The 21ˢᵗ Century Guide to
Writing Articles
in the
Biomedical
Sciences

The 21st Century Guide to
Writing Articles
in the
Biomedical
Sciences

Shiri Diskin
Science Write Right, Israel

W$\ominus$ World Scientific

NEW JERSEY · LONDON · SINGAPORE · BEIJING · SHANGHAI · HONG KONG · TAIPEI · CHENNAI · TOKYO

Published by

World Scientific Publishing Co. Pte. Ltd.

5 Toh Tuck Link, Singapore 596224

USA office: 27 Warren Street, Suite 401-402, Hackensack, NJ 07601

UK office: 57 Shelton Street, Covent Garden, London WC2H 9HE

Library of Congress Cataloging-in-Publication Data

Names: Diskin, Shiri, author.

Title: The 21st century guide to writing articles in the biomedical sciences / Shiri Diskin.

Other titles: Twenty-first century guide to writing articles in the biomedical sciences

Description: Hackensack, NJ : World Scientific, 2018. |
   Includes bibliographical references and index.

Identifiers: LCCN 2017047288| ISBN 9789813231863 (hardcover : alk. paper) |
   ISBN 9813231866 (hardcover : alk. paper) | ISBN 9789813233751 (pbk. : alk. paper) |
   ISBN 9813233753 (pbk. : alk. paper)

Subjects: | MESH: Medical Writing

Classification: LCC R119 | NLM WZ 345 | DDC 808.06/661--dc23

LC record available at https://lccn.loc.gov/2017047288

British Library Cataloguing-in-Publication Data

A catalogue record for this book is available from the British Library.

For any available supplementary material, please visit
http://www.worldscientific.com/worldscibooks/10.1142/10760#t=suppl

Foreword

I have always been passionate about writing, and oddly enough — about scientific writing. I think that communicating science is the number one driver of scientific advancement and hence, perceive knowledge-sharing as the scientist's duty.

At the same time, I can understand how the burdens of everyday life can prevent you, the scientist, from writing. As a professional engaged in biomedical research, especially one for whom research is a pursuit secondary to clinical work, you may be overwhelmed by the sheer number of items on your daily to-do list. Writing becomes a daunting task and is thus postponed, with the hope that in the future, life will be more relaxed and you will have the large blocks of free time that you assume you need in order to get your writing done. When I set out to write this book, I envisioned a reader who is a professional a few years out of school. You, my reader, most likely do not have a very active mentor in your professional life, as was your privilege during your school years. This allows you a greater degree of freedom, but at the same time requires you to make important decisions by yourself.

I assume that you are reading this book because you have conducted research, have acquired data and are now interested in publishing it. In this age of unprecedented flourishing of scientific publishing, when the number and variety of scientific journals are growing daily, (almost) everything is publishable. This should encourage you to write and gain experience in this aspect of the scientific work. Be assured that as long as the work is scientifically sound, it will find its place in the literature.

My aim in this book is to provide practical tools, to reveal to you, my reader, that the huge, overwhelming task of writing a paper is in fact a collection of small, manageable tasks that bear a lot of similarity across different types of papers. Ultimately, I hope to lower the "activation energy" required for initiating the process of writing your paper.

This book is meant for professionals who are writing papers in the biomedical sciences, but many aspects can be applied to other fields as well.

I wish you the best of luck in your writing.

Acknowledgements

My deepest thanks are extended to my loving family, who believed in me, supported me and encouraged me throughout the work on this book.

Contents

1

Before you Write

Chapter 1 in 200 Words for Geniuses

You should keep up-to-date with the literature on an ongoing basis. This can help direct your research, and reduce the need for intense literature searching and reading at the time of initiating your writing process.

1. Set a fixed time for reading in your schedule.
2. Use online "push" services to constantly be updated.
   a. Sign up for newsletters from the leading journals in your field.
   b. Use social media.
   c. Register for a My NCBI account and set up a notification schedule.
3. Be organized, construct a repository for background literature:
   a. On a physical hard-drive or a personal cloud-based folder: Devise a filing system that is easily understandable to you and that allows you to easily recognize the files.
   b. Use citation management software.
   c. Use the feature of a personal library in your My NCBI account.

Understand the level of scientific evidence of the papers you are reading and their importance. Understand how certain papers that you read relate to your work.

Conduct your research ethically, write your paper ethically, including making sure that the list of authors is complete and justifiable in its entirety and disclose all possible conflicts of interest, especially financial ones.

1.1 Keeping Up-to-Date With the Literature

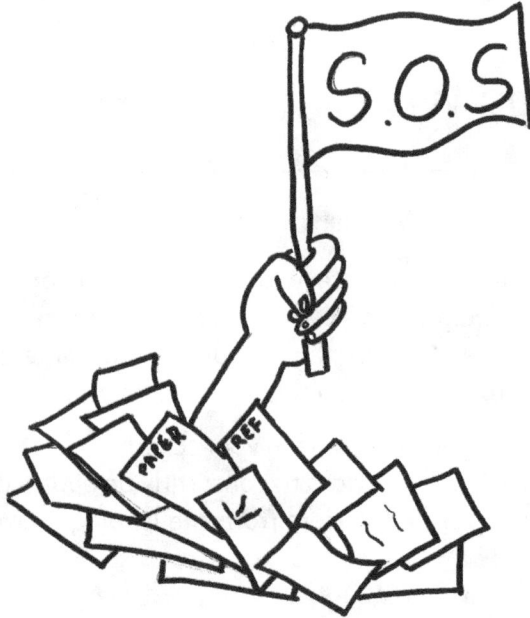

If you keep up-to-date with relevant literature on a continuous basis, you will not start your writing process with an overwhelming reading list.

I do not subscribe to the method of starting the writing process with an intensive reading and studying period. I believe that a much more useful, realistic and less stressful way to go about it is to read on an ongoing basis. This can be of much use to you in planning your research to avoid repeating other people's mistakes or their already published results. If you implement some of the ideas detailed below, when you initiate your writing process, you will already have a rich, well-organized and up-to-date personal library of background materials that you are fairly-well acquainted with. This will leave you with much less left to do in the way of literature searches, that are (from my experience) the most time consuming and exhausting part of writing.

1. Set time for reading. Set a realistic goal that fits your schedule, but strive to meet it regularly.

2. Use online "push" services to constantly be updated.
   a. For general news in your field, sign up for newsletters from the leading journals in your field. You will get the tables of contents (TOC) of the journal every time it is published. Once you receive the TOC, skim the titles of the research articles. Many journals only publish a few (10–20) research articles in each volume. Get into the habit of marking abstracts you want to read. When your scheduled reading time arrives, you will have a pre-selected reading list to start from.
   b. Use social media. At the time of the writing of this book (early 2018), many prominent journals in the fields of medicine (e.g. Lancet[1], JAMA[2], NEJM[3]) and science (e.g. Science[4], Nature[5]) have very active Facebook pages. You can passively get highlights from these publications sent to your Facebook Newsfeed. As you would with any item on your Newsfeed, open select links to read more and e-mail yourself abstracts that seem interesting and/or relevant.
   c. In addition to scientific publishers, a large number of professional societies also maintain active Facebook (e.g. AAAS[6], the American Medical Association[7]) and LinkedIn pages (e.g. AAAS[8], American Medical Association[9]). For the most part, these pages are open to the public; you do not have to be a paying member to get news from these organizations. Another useful method is following interesting pharmaceutical companies on LinkedIn. This can help you learn early of interesting findings that they make in clinical or non-clinical studies. These latter two sources

---

[1] https://www.facebook.com/TheLancetMedicalJournal/
[2] https://www.facebook.com/JAMA-87087958340/
[3] https://www.facebook.com/pages/The-New-England-Journal-of-Medicine/109506135735155
[4] https://www.facebook.com/ScienceMagazine/
[5] https://www.facebook.com/nature/?nr
[6] https://www.facebook.com/AAAS.Science/?nr
[7] https://www.facebook.com/AmericanMedicalAssociation
[8] https://www.linkedin.com/groups/27230/profile
[9] https://www.linkedin.com/company/7077?trk=prof-exp-company-name

of information require extra caution; you cannot use press releases from any of these sources unless they provide a source from a peer-reviewed publication.

d. Register for a My NCBI[10] account. Among many other features, My NCBI allows you to save a specific search. The service e-mails you, on a schedule you define, the updated list of the results of your search, such that you do not miss out on new publications that may be relevant to your work.

3. Read efficiently, mainly abstracts. Choose papers that you deem important and/or interesting to read in full. Try to take note of why you think each paper is important.

4. Understand how certain papers relate to your work. Have you been "scooped"? Has anyone done a similar thing in a different system? With a different method? How do their results affect your hypothesis (if at all)?

5. Be organized, construct a repository for background literature, either physical, or much better, digital. This will come in very handy during the writing process. Consider summarizing in a few points in a constantly updated file what you found interesting in each paper you save/download. My preference for paperless is so strong, that I would rather scan an article and save it digitally than keep a paper copy. With the constantly evolving capabilities of software such as Adobe Acrobat[11] or Foxit PDF[12], you can now highlight text right on a digital Portable Document Format (PDF) file, making paper copies completely redundant.

a. On a physical hard-drive or a personal cloud-based folder: Devise a filing system that is easily understandable to you and that allows you to easily recognize the files. One good method is to use the last name of the first author and the year of publication as the name of the file. Try to come up with a system that will allow you later to remember what was important and why you chose to save certain papers. An example of that could be having a folder in your repository for methods and another for specific

---

[10] https://www.ncbi.nlm.nih.gov/account
[11] https://get.adobe.com/reader/
[12] https://www.foxitsoftware.com/

aspects of the background (for instance a subfolder for the disease you are working on and others for specific therapies).

b. Citation management software such as the free, open-source ZOTERO[13], or the freemium MENDELEY[14] are extremely useful tools for ongoing maintenance of a personal literature collection. With such software, you can download the full and accurate citation directly from Pubmed[15] or Google Scholar[16] into your pre-defined library. If you have a stored full-text copy of the paper, you can link its location on your computer to the citation within your reference library, such that you can open it when you need, directly from within the citation management app, with no need to look for it in your folders. As they both save the Abstract within the citation file, you will easily remember why you originally chose to read a specific paper. In addition, there is the option to add notes to a citation file, allowing you to remind yourself of the specific relevance of the paper to your work.

c. An important feature of the My NCBI account is that it allows you to save citations into collections that you can define and manage within your account. Many Pubmed abstracts have links to full text articles, either in Pubmed Central (PMC) or at the publisher's site. In addition, many academic institutions offer the option to access their online subscriptions directly from within Pubmed through specialized links.

6. Become acquainted with opinion leaders in your field, learn the big names. Understand the publishing landscape — what are the most prominent publications in your field? Familiarity with prominent figures and research groups in your field can help you evaluate the papers that you read and give you a notion of their relative importance, as you use them to analyze your own work.

7. Read Papers in a utilitarian manner, not as you would read a book. What are you trying to learn from the paper? Focus on the section of the paper that is of interest to you and read it first. Then, if you have

---

[13] https://www.zotero.org/

[14] https://www.mendeley.com/

[15] https://www.ncbi.nlm.nih.gov/pubmed

[16] https://scholar.google.com/

not yet done so, re-read the Abstract, look at the figures and tables and at the discussion.

1.2 As You Read, Understand the Levels of Scientific Evidence

The hierarchy of scientific evidence is a concept from the field of evidence-based medicine. Most physicians strive to offer care that is grounded in scientific evidence, but while it is generally accepted that randomized controlled trials (RCTs) are the medical gold standard for support of a medicinal claim, the differences in scientific strength between other types of studies are less obvious. Beginning in the 1980s, various committees around the world have generated rankings of types of studies that serve as a basis for professional guidelines and regulations. Rankings are not uniform, but the differences are very small.

The most often-used ranking system for scientific evidence is that of the Oxford Centre for Evidence-based Medicine[17], a variation on which is offered by the American medical association[18]. A simplified version is provided by the Australian government department of health in this diagram[19].

RCTs are an established standard for evidence-based medicine. Participants in such studies are recruited to achieve a sample that is homogeneous with respect to pre-defined characteristics, and are allocated in a random manner to receive either active therapy, control therapy or placebo. Such studies may employ other design aspects aimed at reducing bias, including masking the treatment assignment from the researcher, from the participant or both.

An even higher level of evidence is a number of RCTs looking at a similar medical question, with similar designs and similar populations.

---

[17] http://www.cebm.net/oxford-centre-evidence-based-medicine-levels-evidence-march-2009/

[18] http://journalofethics.ama-assn.org/2011/01/pfor2-1101.html

[19] https://www.tga.gov.au/sites/default/files/cm-evidence-listed-medicines-05-01.gif

A systematic review of such a group of studies can provide an overview of whether a certain result is strong enough or whether it was unique to a specific study and was not replicated in other studies. The Cochrane reviews are a very good example of a collection of such scientifically-vigorous systematic reviews. Thus, the topmost level of scientific evidence is the systematic review, a subtype of which is the meta-analysis that can provide a quantitative result of the combination of analyzed studies.

Lower in the hierarchy are cohort studies, which tend to form a sizeable proportion of the types of research conducted by younger medical professionals. These are studies in which pre-defined populations are followed over time with the attempt of finding certain parameters that are correlated to a certain outcome. For the most part, such studies are conducted retrospectively, by analyzing medical records and databases containing data that has been collected as part of the patient's routine care. Provided access to the right database, such studies can have the advantage of a very large amount of data spanning many years of follow-up. However, cohort studies can also be conducted in a prospective manner, with the distinct advantage that the data of interest is collected at pre-defined intervals in a uniform manner. Well-controlled and designed case-series, especially those with a relatively large sample, in which each case (patient) has one or more adequate controls, are on a similar level of scientific evidence as cohort studies.

Last, but not least in the hierarchy of levels of scientific evidence are medicinal claims based on the clinical experience and opinions of experts, or on the extrapolation of non-clinical data (*in vitro* studies and/ or animal research).

In your writing, you will need to be aware of these distinctions when writing the Introduction to your papers; to understand which claims have been well-enough supported to form a strong basis for your own work. You would also need to take these definitions into account when writing your Discussion section, when comparing your results with others' in your field.

1.3 Understanding Your Own Research

Either through writing a grant proposal, a study protocol or an Ethics Committee approval request, you must always have a defined research question. What is the gap in current knowledge in the field? What do you (plural — your team, your mentor) think are the possible answers to this question? How is your study going to answer this question? A research question should be very simple and straight forward. You should be able to explain it to an educated person who is a complete layperson in your field.

The logic of the study may be controversial, innovative, "out of the box", but it must be coherent. It is an ethical principle — it is ethically unjustifiable to expose humans or animals or to merely waste resources on research that has no aim. It is also a practical principle — If you cannot explain your research, you cannot get funding for it, nor publish it later. You cannot form collaborations; you cannot hire help or get hired. Science and medicine cannot advance.

1.4 Some Notes on Ethical Conduct

Ethics is sometimes thought of as an intuitive thing. If you are a good and honest person, you probably conduct your research ethically. The reality is that ethics is many times a technical thing. You need to follow the ethical rules set forth by the institution in which you conduct your research, rules that are affected by the rules and regulations of your geographic location (country, state, etc.). However, your target journal and its publisher, may be obliged to follow a different code of ethics than your institution. One example for a publication-specific code of ethics is the ethical standards established by the Committee on Publication Ethics (COPE[20]). Since the biomedical scientific publishing industry is global, the publisher is most likely located in another country, and its code of ethics may be affected by certain cultural or regional sensitivities that differ from your institution's. Thus, it is highly important to

---

[20] https://publicationethics.org/

know what are the specific ethical requirements emphasized by the journal and to make sure that your research not only meets them, but also that the adherence to ethical requirements is well-documented.

Ethical conduct that is relevant to biomedical article publication can be generally divided into 3 main categories, as detailed below.

1.4.1 *Conduct Your Research Ethically*

As a rule — follow your institution's code of ethics. Some important points that should be considered, even if not specifically mentioned in your institution's code include: use adequate controls and appropriate methods and tools (identical and calibrated in the exact same manner for the experimental and control arms of your study). In research involving animals, cause minimal discomfort and suffering to lab animals, use animals as low as possible on the phylogenetic scale and use a justifiable number of animals. In clinical studies, make sure you conduct an adequate procedure of informed consent, recruit a justifiable number of subjects, with a justifiable composition of study population, conduct your study in a manner that minimizes the harm and maximizes the benefit to participants and ensure patient privacy. Crucially: obtain and document approvals from ethics committees for any study involving human or animal subjects.

1.4.2 *Write Your Paper Ethically*

Make sure you present your results ethically (see discussion in Section 4.3). Plagiarism, the use of previously-published ideas or text without attribution, is absolutely forbidden. Today, most scientific publishers use plagiarism-detection software. This type of computer program (e.g. Similarity check by Crossref[21]) compares the text in a submitted manuscript to a large database of published articles, and provides a quantitative output of the degree of textual similarities between the submitted manuscript and previously published papers to editors for further review. It is then up to the editor to decide whether the results are acceptable. Naturally, all scientific work is based on previous science, and thus papers

---

[21] https://www.crossref.org/services/similarity-check/

presenting work in similar fields will likely contain similar background information. The key to making sure your manuscript does not constitute plagiarism is to cite and attribute the source correctly (see Chapter 5).

1.4.3 *Disclose All Possible Conflicts of Interest, Mostly Financial Ones*

It is obvious that research conducted with funding from a commercial entity that stands to benefit from a specific result may constitute a conflict of interests and should be declared. However, other types of conflict, that are more subtle, should also be declared. For instance, if you or any of your co-authors are candidates for a job in the commercial entity, or if a close relative has a vested interest in a publication of a certain result. The International Committee of Medical Journal Editors (ICMJE)[22] provides a comprehensive disclosure form that is required to be signed prior to acceptance of manuscripts in some journals. It is good practice to read this form and ask yourself these questions even when submitting to a journal that does not require it. This way, you can be sure that your disclosure is up to the publishing world's standards.

The matter of authorship is discussed in Section 1.5.

1.5 Some Notes on Choosing Your Co-authors

It is true that you cannot always choose your co-authors. Most research is conducted in hierarchical organizations and it is usually the highest-ranking person in the list of authors, the one whose name appears last, that gets to decide who is named as author and what the order of authors is. Authorship is a matter that is taken gravely seriously within the biomedical-science publishing world. There are basic requirements that have to be met for a person to qualify as an article author. The ICMJE[21] has composed a list of 4 requirements of people who can be considered authors on a paper: Ones who made substantial contributions to the conception or design of the work; or the

---

[22] http://www.icmje.org/

acquisition, analysis, or interpretation of data for the work; AND Drafting the work or revising it critically for important intellectual content; AND Final approval of the version to be published; AND Agreement to be accountable for all aspects of the work in ensuring that questions related to the accuracy or integrity of any part of the work are appropriately investigated and resolved.

However, it has been my experience that researchers of many levels of seniority find themselves pressured to include someone's name on the list of authors of their paper, even if that person did not contribute substantially to the work being reported. There is no simple solution to a situation like that. It is unfair and unethical of anyone to get undue authorship but many times you just want to get your work published and are not up for an ethical crusade. The one suggestion that I may make, is to try and get a meeting with such tacked-on authors, and get them to review the paper. Try to gently force them to contribute to the result-interpretation part of the work. Try to enlist their assistance in discussing your results within a bigger context, assist in choosing a suitable target journal and suggest reviewers.

Considering that journals may contact each author on the list to request their individual approval to publish the paper, make sure that everyone on the list has read the paper, knows where it is submitted for publication and has no objections.

Disputes over authorship are usually dealt with within the academic institutions; however, it is important to know that if you feel that you meet the authorship requirements for a paper that was published without giving you credit, you can contact the journal editor. While not obligated to act on it, a journal may initiate an inquiry. This considered, make sure that you include all deserving authors on the papers under your responsibility.

One final note, professional medical writers such as myself, who have not participated in the conduct of the study or interpretation of results and have been paid for writing or editing the paper, are not automatically considered authors. The codes of ethics of professional associations of medical writers, including the European Medical Writers'

Associations and the American Medical Writers' Association call for medical writers to be acknowledged in the acknowledgement section, in fairness to their effort as well as for the sake of transparency. However, unless they actually meet the above-mentioned requirements for authorship, they should not be included in the list of authors. Recommended best practices for working with professional medical writers can be found in the joint statement of medical writers' organizations ("AMWA–EMWA–ISMPP Joint Position Statement on the Role of Professional Medical Writers" 2017).

2

Choosing your Target Journal

Chapter 2 in 200 Words for Geniuses

You should choose your target journal or journals prior to initiating the writing. Prepare a ranked list of possible target journals, based on the ones you became acquainted with through your ongoing reading, by using journal search engines or through recommendations of senior and experienced colleagues.

The impact factor (IF) is not the only parameter to consider when choosing a target journal. Read the journal's "aims and scope" on the website to understand the degree to which your paper is within the journal's range of topics, how well its audience suits your current paper and the types of articles it publishes (reviews, case reports, etc.).

Take the mode of access (full or partial open-access vs. subscription-based access) into account; understand the fees involved and your ability to pay them.

Read the instructions for authors;

1. Does the journal accept the type of paper that you are planning to write?
2. What are the ethical requirements?
3. What are the formatting instructions?
   a. How many words/tables/figures are allowed?
   b. How many authors can be listed?
   c. What is the required format for citations and bibliographical lists?
   d. What are the technical requirements for figures?
4. Does the journal require adherence to specific reporting guidelines?

Surely there has been a mistake, this should be Chapter 8, right?

In fact, no. The selection of the journal or, more accurately, a few journals to be your submission targets is one of the first steps you need to take, before you initiate the actual writing. The reason for this is that the journal is a crucial determinant of the style and the content of your article. As I have acknowledged before (See Section 1.5), as a scientist making the first steps into article writing, you will likely not be the topmost ranking person in your research group hierarchy and thus will have to consult with more senior colleagues about the correct journal for submission. Be that as it may, informed participation in the decision-making process will provide you with a higher chance of affecting it.

2.1 What Can We Learn from the Journal's "Aims and Scope"?

2.1.1 *Topics, Article Types and Readership*

Everyone is familiar with the Thomson-Reuters impact factor (IF)[1]. There is a notion among scientists that one should "aim as high as possible" on the IF scale. The IF of the journal in which a paper is published, is perceived as a direct measure of the quality and importance of the paper itself and of the researcher's work in general. However, the truth is a bit more complicated than that. A journal and a manuscript are, in many ways, similar to a job and a candidate. Each one of them has a complex set of considerations that makes the other a better (or worse) match.

The current era in the history of biomedical publishing is characterized by an ever-growing number of journals. As a researcher, you are faced with the dilemma of where to submit your paper for publication. The better the match between your manuscript and the journal, the higher the chances of it getting accepted. The first things to know about a journal you are considering for your paper, are its aims and scope. These could generally be found on the journal's website, to varying levels of

---

[1] http://ipscience.thomsonreuters.com/product/journal-citation-reports/?utm_source=false&utm_medium=false&utm_campaign=false#

detail. The information usually includes the areas of research that are published in the journal and whether it is focused on clinical applications or basic sciences. On the journal's website, within its "aims and scope" or "about" tabs, you will most likely find a general description of the target audience (e.g. nurses, geneticists, veterinarians, surgeons). This information may include statements about the journal being an official publication of a professional association/society, which is an additional way to understand the degree to which its audience suits your current paper. The narrower the focus of the journal, the more likely you are to see specific topics that the journal does not cover, and will not publish. You will also find information regarding the types of articles it publishes (original research, reviews, case studies, methods/protocols and others).

2.1.2 *Mode of Access*

A very important piece of information is the mode of access. Journals today operate in one of two major business models: the traditional pay-wall model and the open-access (OA) model. Both models include a small processing fee prior to acceptance. Under the traditional model, the reader (or the institution) pays a fee for access to the full text of a published article. This can be per-article or as part of a subscription. The OA model is reversed, the author pays a publication fee for the accepted article, and any reader can access the full text of the article for free. Full free access can be immediate (Gold open access) or the article may become freely available following an embargo period (Green open access) (Frank 2013). Under the OA model, article processing fees (APC), can run as high as thousands of dollars in some journals[2]. OA journals list their publication fees on their websites. If the funding body or your institution will not reimburse you for APCs, and your institution does not hold a membership for the journal that includes a partial fee waiver, make sure you can afford the APC out of pocket. There are a few other options for authors with limited funds. Some publishers offer full and partial waiver programs. Some large publishing houses (including

---

[2] http://www.lib.berkeley.edu/scholarlycommunication/oa_fees.html

SpringerOpen and BioMed Central[3], Wiley[4] and Elsevier[5]) give priority for fee waivers or even automatic fee waivers to authors based in countries eligible for research4life[6] access. Certain professional societies that publish OA journals may sometimes fund, fully or partially the OA costs of certain papers.

2.1.3 *Editorial Board and Journal Metrics*

In some journals, you will see information about the number of issues per year, which can impact the time to publication (see Section 2.3), and in some cases, a wider range of metrics, including an estimated turnaround time from submission to acceptance, the average number of downloads, IF and other rankings. The names of the editor-in-chief and the editorial board can also be found on the website. This information may be of some importance in the choice of submission target; for instance, it is valuable to know whether any of your co-authors is or works closely with a journal's board member.

An important detail to look for is the indexing services that list the journal. The range of indexing services around the world is wide, but for papers in the biomedical sciences, my personal preference has always been to avoid publication in journals that are not listed on Medline/Pubmed (see Section 5.1).

2.2 A Note on "Predatory Journals"

Predatory journals are commercial enterprises that exploit the principles of OA scientific publishing to make a profit. Like legitimate OA journals, they charge authors a fee for publishing their work. Unlike legitimate OA journals, they employ little to no oversight on the content of the published papers, and provide no editorial services or quality control. The

---

[3] https://www.springer.com/gp/open-access/open-access-funding
[4] http://www.wileyopenaccess.com/details/content/13707a1ddf6/Waivers-and-Discounts-on-Article-Publication-Charges.html
[5] https://www.elsevier.com/about/company-information/policies/pricing)
[6] http://www.research4life.org/eligibility/

term was coined by an American librarian, Jeffrey Beall, who, until January 2017 maintained a list of publishers that he deemed potential, possible, or probable predatory scholarly OA publishers. The list was met with a lot of support, as well as criticism and was recently un-published. The main difference between legitimate and non-legitimate scientific journals, is the level of responsibility they assume on the content that they publish, and that has a lot to do with the editorial board. Legitimate journals employ review and assessment procedures on the papers that they publish and whether or not they enlist the assistance of peer-reviewers, ultimately, the decision on whether to publish a paper lies with the editor (see Section 9.1).

Predatory journals hurt the scientific community in a few ways: as a scientist, you cannot rely on the information they provide as background for your own research; as an author, publishing in such a journal is a waste of a lot of work and money, as this type of publication may not account toward fulfilling the criteria for career advancement or for funding opportunities, and the lack of professional review deprives you, the author, of valuable scientific input.

In a broader sense, these publications undermine the status of science in the view of the general public and that may have dire consequences.

What can you do? Be vigilant. As a reader and an author of scientific publications, inspect the source before using or disseminating information. If you are not yet an established "name" in your field, there is probably no real reason for a journal to solicit papers from you (or, for that matter, invite you to speak at conferences). Consider any such invitation to be spam and discard it. Use verified indexes (see Section 5.1) to assess any journal prior to submitting anything to it for publication or citing any of its papers. For biomedical work, my preference has always been and continues to be the use of Pubmed as the search engine of choice, relying heavily on the vetting process employed by the American National Library of Medicine to weed out less trustworthy publications from my reading lists.

It has recently been announced that the Beall list will be re-published, this time as a continually-updated commercial database of journals and publishers under the auspices of PubsHub[7]. This would become a searchable and thus, very useful resource for researchers trying to assess a journal prior to submitting a manuscript.

2.3 Define Your Publication Goals and Prepare a Ranked List of Publication Targets

Papers are almost never published in the first journal they are submitted to. As you gain more experience, it will become easier for you to identify a journal that is more likely to accept your paper and avoid repeated rounds of submission and revision with different journals.

When you write a paper, you need to know what your goals are in the short- and long-term. Are you up for a new position? Submitting a grant proposal? About to change focus in your research and need to reach out to a new community of researchers? Are you trying to affect policy or legislation? Are you marketing anything? Are you interested in a journal that publishes very fast? A journal that garners a lot of exposure (including exposure to the general-public)? The answers to each of these questions (and others) will help you understand what emphasis you should put on specific journal parameters.

2.3.1 *Study Topic and Field of Research*

You want to publish your research in a journal within your field, but what is your field? Consider, for example, a retrospective analysis of children's medical records aimed at finding risk factors for developing diabetes before age 18. This type of research can be suitable for a pediatrics journal, an endocrinology journal, a pediatric endocrinology journal, a diabetes journal, a pediatric diabetes journal and depending on the results, maybe for a wide variety of public-health-policy journals. Thus, field of study is only a very crude criterion by which to make a preliminary attempt at narrowing down the list of possible submission targets.

---

[7]http://www.pubshub.com/

2.3.2 *Online Journal-Selecting Search Engines*

Because you are up-to-date with your reading (see Section 1.1), you already know which journals publish the articles that are of the most interest to you. You can decide to create a list of submission targets from within this group of journals and you can also use online journal-selecting search engines. Major publishers provide free search engines that can help in selecting a target journal from their catalogue. To use these engines, you need a general description of the research or a list of key concepts. You can paste one of these into the search box of the Elsevier[8] or Springer[9] search engines, or use the general free search engines JournalGuide[10] or sjfinder[11] that are not affiliated with a specific publisher. Each of these engines employs a different algorithm, but the output from the search is usually a list of journals rated by a "match index" with information about the IF, mode of access, publishing speed and more. In my opinion, you should run your search on multiple engines, and add your own favorite journals to the list. Online journal selecting search engines offer a filter that can exclude all OA journals (see Section 2.1.2) from your search results, but I do not recommend this strategy. Find out the actual cost of publication in a specific journal and your available funding options, before foregoing the advantages of publication under the OA model.

2.3.3 *Time to Publication*

Be aware that you cannot set a deadline for the actual publication, as the process is long and involves steps that are unpredictable, including the scope of changes suggested by reviewers and the time it will take you to implement them (see Section 9.4). You can get some direct and indirect information about the typical time it takes a journal to return comments from reviewers and to publish a manuscript after it has been accepted. As

---

[8] http://journalfinder.elsevier.com/
[9] http://www.springer.com/gp/authors-editors/journal-author/journal-author-helpdesk/preparation/1276#c1258
[10] https://www.journalguide.com/
[11] http://www.sjfinder.com/journals/recommend

I mentioned, for some journals, such statistics are provided on the website and this information may even appear in the journal selector output. For others, there sometimes is information on Pubmed, concerning date of submission and date of publication per specific papers. The number of issues per year is a good indication of speed; however, today most journals publish papers online prior to printing them (see Section 9.6.4), and for most purposes, this online pre-publication is the date that "counts" and the volume/issue exact citation is of less importance.

As I said, the first journal to which you submit your paper is very rarely the one that you end up publishing in. As discussed in Section 9.5, if your paper needs to be submitted to a different journal, you will need to identify another, potentially more suitable target journal, revise your paper and go through the whole submission process. Publishers offer a service to help you bypass this ordeal. Upon rejection of your paper from one journal, you will be offered the option to send your paper to the transfer service (see examples at Elsevier[12] and at Springer[13]). The staff there can analyze your paper and offer you one or more of the same publisher's journals as alternative targets for resubmission. In some cases, you may also add your own ideas for target journals to the list, as long as they are from the same publisher. You can then approve for them to resubmit your paper, without any need for you to revise it, to the newly-chosen journal, usually accompanied by the reviewers' comments. This service is very useful and a good time saver. Seeing as you retain the final decision on the new target journal, I see no reason to decline the option afforded by this service.

If you need to reach a wide audience beyond your research field community, or if you need to reach the general-public, you should choose journals that publicize papers in social media, press releases, newsletters etc.

After you have generated a list of approximately 10 journals that are suitable in terms of price of publication, research topic and type of paper, rank them for yourself in terms of speed of publication and spe-

---

[12] https://www.elsevier.com/authors/journal-authors/submit-your-paper/submit-and-revise/article-transfer-service

[13] https://www.springer.com/gp/authors-editors/journal-author/the-springer-transfer-desk

cific target audience. As a last means of ranking, use the IF and among the journals that are best suited for your goals, aim as high as you can.

2.4 Informed Reading of the Journal's Guidelines for Authors

As I mentioned at the top of this chapter, the journal you are going to submit to will affect the content, as well as the format of your paper. In most cases, you will find instructions for authors (sometimes called "submission guidelines") on the journal's website[14]. There are some journals that provide instructions for authors within the online submission system whose services they use[15]. Note that some journals have two sets of instructions, one within the journal's website and one within the online-submission website; thus, it is always a good idea to check both places. Unfortunately, there are some journals for which the instructions in those two places are contradictory. If you are confident that you have identified a contradiction, try to contact the editorial office via mail or phone call to get clarification on which set of instructions applies. If, for any reason, you are unable to get a definitive answer to such a query, follow the instruction on the submission system, as many times the system will automatically prevent you from submitting papers that do not adhere to its instructions (see Section 8.7).

The level of detail into which the instructions delve, varies greatly between journals, and has a lot to do with the professional discipline. There are some core issues that generally appear in all sets of instructions for authors:

1. The types of papers that are accepted. Read this section carefully, especially when your paper is something other than a full research paper. A few examples include:

    •   If you are writing a review, make sure the journal accepts unsolicited reviews.

---

[14] See Example in: https://bmcinfectdis.biomedcentral.com/submission-guidelines
[15] See example in: http://edmgr.ovid.com/pain/accounts/ifauth.htm instructions for authors submitting to PAIN journal within the Editorial Manager® website.

- If you are writing a short paper to report a small number of results, make sure the journal publishes "short communications" or "research briefs".
- If you intend to write a case report, make sure the journal publishes case reports and whether there are specific requirements for a case to merit publication of a case report. Some journals will only publish very specific, innovative, cutting-edge cases or ones with a specific application, such as a new surgical technique.
- If you are trying to publish a study protocol, it may be a little harder to find a journal that would publish it, so read instructions carefully before you submit.

2. The ethical requirements (see Section 1.4).

3. Copyright issues. When you publish your paper in a journal under the traditional pay-wall model, your copyrights for the published materials, including illustrations, pictures, etc. are transferred to the journal. You need to read the section regarding copyrights carefully, because if you expect to need to use these materials in the future (for instance, as part of a book chapter or a review article you write), you may need to obtain permission from the publisher to use your own materials that you have published. In OA journals, you retain the copyright and can use the materials freely, but (provided integrity is maintained and your work is properly cited) so can everyone else[16] (See also Section 9.6).

4. Formatting instructions. Meeting the journal's technical requirements is of high importance, because in the review process, this is the first thing that is checked (see Section 9.1), and if your paper does not meet the requirements, you will lose valuable time when it gets sent back to you without even being reviewed for content. So, prior to writing, understand what the journal requires of you and prepare your manuscript accordingly right from the start. If you are submitting your paper to a second journal following a rejection, be sure to adjust formatting to meet the new journal's requirements (also see Section 9.5). The formatting instructions section varies

---

[16] http://www.openoasis.org/index.php%3Foption%3Dcom_content%26view%3Darticle%26id%3D550%26Itemid%3D372

greatly in the level of detail between journals. Some journals provide sparse instructions that tell you in very general terms, only the number of pages that a paper of a certain type can span[17]. More detailed instructions may, for example, specify the number of words allowed for the Abstract and number of words allowed for the entire text, any limit on number of authors, number and technical requirements of visual aids (see Section 4.5), the formatting of in-text citations and the bibliographical list (see Section 5.5), and requirements for availability of raw data (see Section 4.5)[18].

One of the big publishing houses, Elsevier, has a program called "your paper your way"[19], which allows you to initially submit a paper in any reasonable format that allows a reviewer to assess the content of the manuscript, and imposes formatting requirements only at later stages. This provides flexibility that can be translated into speed. If your paper is rejected by a journal, you can submit it to another without much revision that is aimed solely at adjusting the formatting to meet the new journal's requirements.

5. Reporting Guidelines. Some journals require authors to adhere to specific reporting guidelines, and to provide proof, in the form of a checklist or a flow-chart. Some examples of reporting guidelines that are applicable to certain types of biomedical research are Consolidated Standards of Reporting Trials (CONSORT), which refer mainly to RCTs[20] and other guidelines curated by the EQUATOR network[21] that span the gamut of clinical and non-clinical studies. Make sure you know which guidelines are required for your type of study by your target journal and that your manuscript adheres to the guideline. This will be useful even if you are rejected and need to re-submit to another journal without this requirement, as the guidelines are very helpful in constructing clear and transparent manuscripts.

---

[17] See example, website of the Journal of Attention Disorders https://uk.sagepub.com/en-gb/mst/journal-of-attention-disorders/journal201756#submission-guidelines

[18] See example, website of Emergency Medicine Journal http://journals.bmj.com/site/authors/preparing-manuscript.xhtml

[19] https://www.elsevier.com/authors/journal-authors/your-paper-your-way

[20] http://www.consort-statement.org/

[21] http://www.equator-network.org/

3

The Methods Section

Chapter 3 in 200 Words for Geniuses

The Methods section is intended to serve as a type of a recipe, be transparent but do not over elaborate. Make use of the online-only supplementary materials option.

The Methods section should be divided into sub-sections, one for each experiment or data acquisition method. The order of the sub-sections should correspond to the order of result presentation.

Use metric units for height, weight, and volume, degrees Celsius for temperature and mmHg for blood pressure. Laboratory measurements should be reported in SI. Drugs, devices and other products should be mentioned in their nonproprietary names. It is important to use consistent and accurate names for all genes and proteins mentioned in the text.

Provide enough details about the animals used in your research, justify the sample size, and detail any treatment they underwent in the study.

For clinical research (either prospective or retrospective), provide detailed eligibility criteria and justify the sample size. Explain the nature, timing and mode of any intervention, and the exact information you collected in the study. Provide details about any questionnaires you used, including the setting in which they were filled, and how scores were analyzed.

Mention Ethics Committee approval, any measures to ensure participant safety, comfort and privacy and the informed consent procedure (when relevant).

3.1 How Much to Elaborate

The Methods section is intended to serve as a type of a recipe. It should provide enough information to allow the reader, assuming he/she has the required resources, to repeat the authors' work in the exact same manner they performed it. This does not mean that you should write a lengthy tome describing every minute detail of your work. Only new methods should be described in full. Do not over elaborate on well-established routine procedures; just point out the specifics. If you used a commercial kit, state that you have used it per manufacturer's instructions. Published methods, including ones described in your group's previous publications, can be referenced. If you have modified the referenced methods, you should say *"XX was performed as described in [xxx] with the following modifications"*, and list the modifications. It is many times appropriate to explain the reason for the modifications. If you have veered way off of the referenced method, you can say *"the xx procedure was adapted from [xxx]"*.

When applicable, make use of the online-only supplementary materials option. This may be appropriate, among many other options, for lists of gene primers or antibodies and for detailed technical explanations on imaging or other medical devices. You can also present full questionnaires (see Sections 3.5 and 3.7) or detailed descriptions of a unique image analysis method as supplementary materials.

3.2 Writing Style for the Methods Section

3.2.1 *Sub-sections*

The Methods section should be divided into sub-sections, one for each experiment or data acquisition method. The order of the sub-sections should correspond to the order of result presentation (see Chapter 4). Always dedicate a separate sub-section to the statistical methods.

3.2.2 *Tense and Voice*

The Methods section of an article should be written in the past tense; after all, you are describing things that you have done in the past. My personal stylistic preference for the Methods section is the passive English voice: I prefer "Samples were collected" to "we have taken the samples." However, you had better not use passive English if you are not confident in your ability to construct the sentences correctly.

If you choose to write in active English, do not use the first-person singular; it is never "I" who had performed the experiments, but it can be "we". For one thing, this does not sound sophisticated or professional and for another, you are highly unlikely to be the sole author of a published article. You can learn a lot about specific terms, phrases and sentence structures appropriate for the Methods section from Unit 2 of the book *Science Research Writing for Non-Native Speakers of English* (Glasman-Deal 2009).

3.2.3 *Units*

Unless specified otherwise in your target journal's instructions for authors (see Section 2.4), use units as recommended by the ICMJE[1]: metric units for height, weight, and volume (meter, kilogram and liter), temperature in degrees Celsius and blood pressure in millimeters of mercury (mmHg). Laboratory measurements, including hematologic, clinical chemistry and others, should be reported in SI (from French: *Système international d'unités*) units[2]; however it may be appropriate to provide the results in the units originally provided by your lab along with the ones converted to SI. The American Medical Association Manual of Style provides a very user-friendly converter[3]. Standard units of measurement are not considered abbreviations and, unless it is specifically required by the journal, there is no need to spell-out the term upon its first appearance, as you would with other abbreviations.

3.2.4 *Nomenclature*

Drugs, devices and other products should be mentioned in their nonproprietary names, apart from cases in which the trade name is pertinent to

---

[1] http://icmje.org/recommendations/browse/manuscript-preparation/preparing-for-submission.html#j

[2] https://en.wikipedia.org/wiki/International_System_of_Units#Base_units

[3] http://www.amamanualofstyle.com/page/si-conversion-calculator

the topic of the study (for example, when the study is a comparison of the same product by different manufacturers, or if the study is an assessment of a new product belonging to a class of products already on the market). If the substance has a few different names or was once known by a different name, then this should be noted in the text.

It is important to use the correct and accurate names for all genes and proteins mentioned in the text. Be sure to use the same nomenclature consistently throughout the text of your article. The HUGO Gene nomenclature committee website provides a vast catalogue of approved names for human loci, including protein coding genes, ncRNA genes and pseudogenes[4]. They also keep a constantly-updated list of other resources, including databases for non-human genomes, protein bioinformatics and other bioinformatic resources[5]. The national center for Biotechnology Style Guide[6] recommends italicizing genes, but not proteins. Unlike units, gene names should be spelled out in full upon their first appearance in the text, thereafter to be referred to by their abbreviation. Always look for detailed instructions on nomenclature in the journal. In addition, look for articles published recently in your target journal that deal with your gene, and implement their nomenclature of choice. If the gene has many names and specifically, if you are citing previous publications that refer to your gene with different names, make sure to note that in your text ("*previously known as/previously called XXX*").

3.3 Research Involving Animals

Any scientist using living organisms in research should be able to justify the use of those organisms. This is a scientific principle that compels researchers to understand the experimental system in which they work, its advantages and limitations and suitability for addressing the research question. It provides transparency and allows peers to critically-assess the results in the context of the system in which they were obtained.

---

[4] http://www.genenames.org/
[5] http://www.genenames.org/useful/all-links
[6] https://www.ncbi.nlm.nih.gov/books/NBK995/

Moreover, this is an ethical principle. Subjection of animals to experimental procedures should only be done in a justifiable manner, for the sake of answering worthwhile scientific questions that cannot be answered with other, life-sparing approaches.

In 2011, the American National Research Council's Institute for Laboratory Animal Research (ILAR) has published Guidance for the Description of Animal Research in Scientific Publications (National Research Council (US) Institute for Laboratory Animal Research 2011). The guidance, which is freely available online[7] is an important read, especially for scientists making their first steps into publishing papers involving animal research. Here, I list a few details that you should include in your Methods section, according to the guidance.

You should specify the genus and species of the animal and provide details about the age, sex, weight, and life stage of your animals. You should understand, and explain (or reference a previous publication with an explanation) why the specific animal is suitable for the study of your research question and why you chose it at the specific life stage (for example, mouse embryos can provide information on biological processes that geriatric mice cannot).

As with any other resource used in the study, the source from which laboratory animals were obtained should be stated in the paper. This allows any reader who wishes to repeat your experimental design, to obtain animals as close as possible to the ones you used. Other important specifications include the genetic nomenclature and/or the microbial/pathogen status.

The description of your study design should detail the preparation of animals to be included in the study and their assignment to groups (including control groups). This should include the sample size justification.

As part of the ethical conduct and transparency, details about animal husbandry, such as animal environment, diet, water and housing should be provided.

---

[7] https://www.ncbi.nlm.nih.gov/pubmed/22379656

In addition, the Methods section of the article should contain basic animal methodology, including aspects of animal care and use that can affect research outcomes, with detailed information about: any administered treatments (or exposure to infectious agents), methods for collecting samples, measures to minimize suffering (such as anesthesia) and euthanasia.

While you may be required to provide statements about the ethical approval of your study on your Title Page or in a separate document, you should include such a statement in the Methods section of the text as well. Be sure to have documentation for such approval, in case the journal requests it.

3.4 Prospective Clinical Research

3.4.1 *Study Protocol*

Prospective clinical studies are based on clinical study protocols. When writing a paper describing such a study, you have the advantage of the protocol as an information source, that you can adapt to suit the length and level of detail appropriate for a journal article. This is not merely a useful tool, be sure that your article describes the methods as they were performed in actuality, which should be exactly as described in the latest version of the protocol. If this is not the case, you need to mention it, explain the reasons for the deviation and note whether the change was approved by the Ethics Committee. In accordance with journal requirements, you may need to post your study protocol to a publicly-accessible database, such as Clinical trials.gov[8].

3.4.2 *Study Design and Population*

The first paragraph in the Methods section of a paper describing clinical research, should be the study design. Examples of study designs are: parallel, cross-over, randomized, etc. In the Oxford Handbook of Clinical and Healthcare Research (Ray *et al.*, 2016), the authors provide a good

---

[8] https://clinicaltrials.gov/

and thorough primer on the various types of clinical studies and what are the best uses for each type of design.

When describing clinical research, it is of the utmost importance to describe the study population in detail. You should present any inclusion/exclusion criteria and when these criteria go beyond demographics and diagnostic criteria, you should explain the reasoning behind them. For instance, if you have chosen to exclude people who have had treatment with a certain type of drug up to a certain point in time prior to the initiation of your study, this may need explaining. Other types of exclusion criteria may also sometimes require explanations, such as specific age limitations in studies involving pediatric populations (a study conducted only on children between the ages of 8–15, requires reasoning). Specific notice should be taken with regards to the exclusion criteria pertaining to ethnic groups. If you choose to exclude a specific ethnic group from your study, this may amount to an ethical issue and should be discussed with your Ethics Committee.

3.4.3 *Procedures and Research Tools*

In papers describing clinical studies, it is important to explain the nature, timing and mode of any intervention. This may sometimes be best presented in the form of a diagram or a flow chart. The setting in which the intervention was performed is also important (such as a hospital, a clinic, at the patient's home, etc.). The sample size chosen for the study should be justified in the statistical methods paragraph. In any study that has more than a single arm, it is important to describe, and sometimes explain, the differences between the arms, and how this pertains to the study design.

You should be able to explain how the data you collected in the study is the correct choice for answering the research question. Be well-acquainted with the study tools you used; were any procedures meant as safety-data collection? Which of them was an efficacy-assessment measure?

What measures were used to avoid bias? In double-blinded (double-masked) studies, how was the treatment assignment kept concealed from study personnel?

For certain types of studies, such as imaging studies, studies involving surgical interventions and other types of studies whose results can be affected by the proficiency of the person performing the procedures or interpreting their results, it is important to note whether any steps were taken to avoid inter-rater or inter-performer differences. So, for example, you may write "*All surgeries were performed by the same team of surgeons, all experts in the field of XXX*", "*ECG records for all patients during all study visits were interpreted centrally by the same investigator, who was not informed of the identity of the patient or their treatment/placebo assignment*".

Some information may not need to be detailed in full, but you need to have it, in case asked by the journal: What steps did you take to ensure patient safety, comfort and privacy? How was informed consent obtained?

3.5 Retrospective Medical Record Studies

3.5.1 *Data Source*

If you write an article reporting an analysis of data mined from databases, such as retrospective patient records, you should dedicate some text to the description of the data source. It is important to understand whether the data was derived from a computerized database. If so, when have computerized records started? It may sometimes be appropriate to mention how the data were originally obtained. There is a difference between patient records containing data gathered by medical personnel and records based on patients' self-reports. Consider, for example, a study that looks at parameters that may possibly be correlated to a patient's Body Mass Index (BMI). It is important to note whether the patients' weight and height records were based on self-reports or on measurements taken at the clinic.

Descriptions of the data source should include its limitations, for instance, whether some data for certain patients is missing, and whether this affected the analyses. It may be that you decide to include only patients for which the full data set was available. Consider, for example, a retrospective analysis of files of patients who were followed for 10 years. It is very likely that some patients were lost to follow-up after less than 10 years. What did you do with these patients? Did you exclude them from the analysis? Included the data that was available for them? You should clearly define in the Methods section what was the study policy with respect to missing data.

3.5.2 *Ethical Approval and Data Collection Procedure*

In this type of study, it is important to mention whether ethics approval was obtained, or possibly a waiver. It is also very important to explain how patient privacy was maintained.

When conducting a data mining study, whether in paper files or in large digital databases, you should have a pre-defined set of parameters that you collect and record, and this list should be included in the paper's Methods section. It is important in such studies to collect the data in a structured manner, such as with a questionnaire that the data collector fills out for each patient based on the patient's records. If you prepare such a questionnaire, it is valuable to include it as supplementary online-only material. For your own sake, it is important for you to understand the relative importance of each part of the data that you collected and its role within the study's general scientific question. This will help you inter- pret your results, and facilitate the writing of the Discussion.

3.6 Systematic Literature Reviews and Meta Analyses

A publishable systematic literature review is different from a review article. Writing a review article is similar to writing the Introduction of a research paper. You conduct literature searches and dig deeply into the field of knowledge, many times letting the content or references of a paper lead you to your next reading target (see Chapter 5).

A systematic literature review is different[9]. When conducting a system- atic review of literature, you ask a specific question before you start. For

---

[9] ResearchCORE.org

instance: "Is this therapy effective for this indication?" You then design the study and pre-define its methodology, including:

1. The databases to be searched
2. The terms to use in the search
3. Criteria for inclusion of publications in the analysis (e.g. publication years, types of publications [exclude case reports, exclude non-clinical research, exclude conference abstracts], publication languages).

Finally, you conduct the searches, identify the publications that adhere to your inclusion criteria, and conduct your analysis with the aim of answering your pre-defined research question. When you write a paper reporting a systematic review, all the above-mentioned aspects of your study design should be included in the Methods section.

The Cochrane reviews[10] are a prime example of scientifically-rigorous systematic reviews. If you are just starting out in the field of writing systematic reviews, you can use the Cochrane Handbook[11] to learn how to design a systematic review study and report the results.

A "meta-analysis" is a statistical approach to combining the data derived from a systematic-review. In a paper describing a meta-analysis, you should include, in addition to the search aspects of the study design, the statistical analysis used to derive a quantitative result of the combination of analyzed studies.

3.7 Studies Involving Questionnaires

When you write a paper reporting on a study that involved the use of questionnaires, it is very important to provide details about the questionnaire:

- Has the questionnaire been used before? If so, provide references to the original development work. If the current paper is the first publication of the use of this questionnaire, you should describe what

---

[10] http://www.cochranelibrary.com/cochrane-database-of-systematic-reviews/index.html

[11] http://handbook.cochrane.org/

measures were taken to validate it (development of a research questionnaire may sometimes merit a separate paper, see Section 4.2). Did you run a pilot with the questionnaire?

- What research question is the questionnaire meant to answer?

  For example: "*The Conner's Parent Rating Scale —Revised: Short Form (CPRS-R:S)* (Conners, 1997) *is a standard measure used to profile Attention Deficit Hyper Activity symptoms*".

- Is the questionnaire addressed at the study participant (a self-assessment tool, sometimes referred to as "patient-reported-outcome"), at the non-medical caregiver (such as a parent or a spouse) or at their physician?

  Example: "*Patients' health-related quality of life (HrQoL) was assessed using self-reported and caregiver-rated generic (EuroQoL Instrument) and dementia-specific (Quality of Life-Alzheimer's Disease [Qol-AD]) scales*"(Hessmann *et al.*, 2016).

- How many questions are included in the questionnaire? Are they divided into parts/ domains/ modules?

  For example: "*The Movement Disorder Society (MDS)–sponsored revision of the Unified Parkinson's Disease Rating Scale (UPDRS), known as the MDS-UPDRS, comprises four parts: I, Nonmotor Experiences of Daily Living; II, Motor Experiences of Daily Living; III, Motor Examination; and IV, Motor Complications*"(Goetz *et al.*, 2007).

- Are the responses free-text? Multiple choice? Given on a scale?

- If a scale is used, is it an ordinal (Likert[12]) scale or a visual analog scale (VAS[13])?

  Example: "*Items were scored on a 5-point Likert scale (1=always, 5=never)*".

  Example: "*Pain was scored on a 100 mm VAS scale*"

- How is the score calculated? Are there sub-scores for each module? Note that standard assessment tools have published and accepted ways of score analysis, which you should adhere to, unless you can provide very solid reasoning for deviating from them.

- Are there clinically-meaningful score cutoffs?

---

[12] https://en.wikipedia.org/wiki/Likert_scale
[13] https://com-jax-emergency-pami.sites.medinfo.ufl.edu/files/2015/03/Visual-Analog-Scale-VAS-in-depth.pdf

For example: "*The possible range of raw scores on the total scale is 38–190, with higher scores, (155–190) reflecting normal performance. A score of 142–154 reflects a probable difference in performance, while a score of 38–141 reflects a definite difference in performance (Dunn, 1999).*"

It is also very important to explain the setting and methodology of administering the questionnaire:

- Who filled out the questionnaire?
  Did the researcher or the participant fill out the forms? Were the questionnaires paper- or computer- based?
- How were language issues addressed?
  In what language was the questionnaire administered? Was language proficiency part of the inclusion criteria? How were the study participants who are not proficient in the language of the questionnaire assisted? Were interpreters available to assist at the location of the study?
  Was literacy taken into account? How were illiterate participants (including children) assisted?
- What was the setting in which the questionnaire was filled?
  Were the questionnaires filled out at the doctor's office? In a separate room dedicated for the study? At the hospital bedside? In a location chosen by the participant? How may the environmental conditions at the time of questionnaire-filling have affected responses?
  In some cases, the time of week or day may also be relevant information to present as part of the conditions.
- How, and by whom, was informed consent obtained? How were vulnerable populations (such as children, the critically-ill or mentally-disabled) treated with respect to consent to participate in the study?

3.8 Case Reports and Case Series

The case report is one of the basic and most important types of medical information to be shared by clinicians and can be of extreme value during the process of making treatment decisions in non-routine cases.

Medical professionals at the early stages of their career, can benefit from writing case reports. This is good practice and a relatively easy way of starting out as an author. However, you should be aware that some academic institutions do not include case reports in the total count of publications required for obtaining teacher statuses in medical schools (Aggarwal *et al.*, 2016).

When you choose a case to report, you should define for yourself what makes it interesting. It may be that the diagnosis is very rare or unique with respect to the patient's demographic characteristics (consider, for example, a diagnosis of Alzheimer's disease in an 18-year-old patient). It may be that a new imaging modality or surgical procedure was used successfully in a patient or a known therapy adjusted to treat a new indication or a new type of patient.

Presentation of a single case should include demographic information about the patient, the presentation at the initial interaction with the healthcare system, and any relevant background information, including known medical history, co-morbidities, potentially relevant use of medications and medical devices and relevant medical/surgical procedures.

The Methods section of a case report should include all diagnostic, medical or surgical procedures utilized during the management of the case. In this section, write the important procedures, and any procedure that is the routine for management of such a case can just be included in the general statement: "*Vital signs, blood tests and physical examinations were performed as per the hospital's standard of care*". The outcomes at the end of the reported follow-up period and any detail in the management that could potentially have affected the outcome, should be pointed out. You should focus on the aspects of the case that make it of interest and that have led you to write about it.

If you are describing more than one case, each case can be described in less detail. You should emphasize the shared characteristics of the cases, that led you to compile them and present them together. If the patients are related, the type of familial relationship should be noted, and you should consider presenting a family tree. In addition to their similarities, provide information about their differences, specifically those that potentially affect the outcomes. It is almost always appropriate to compare the characteristics of your current case, to previously-published similar cases and to note their similarities and differences, again, with specific emphasis on anything that can be hypothesized to have affected the outcomes.

4

The Results Section

Chapter 4 in 200 Words for Geniuses

The Results section is a presentation of results with no interpretation. As a first step, evaluate your results and understand how well they come together to answer your research question. Do they all support the same conclusion? If there are discrepancies, can they be explained?

Assess how many papers you have; you may sometimes have enough results for more than one paper; at other times, an innovative methodology may merit a separate paper.

The Results section of the article should be divided into subsections, preferably, each containing the answer to one of the scientific sub-questions. The first sub-section will almost always be a description of the actual sample used in the study (human participants/ experimental animals/ reviewed papers, etc.).

The text should be used to provide an overview of the results, point out the most important findings presented in each visual aid and lead the reader through the logical flow of the entire study. Do not reiterate the information presented in visual aids; always cross-reference clearly. Figures and tables should be understandable on their own, with no need to consult the text.

Adhere to the journal's instructions for authors. Write in the past tense and use short sentences. Write your paper ethically with respect to presentation of controls, image manipulation and original source materials.

4.1 Reviewing Your Results, Are You There Yet?

The first thing you need to do when contemplating writing a paper, is review your results. You should critically-assess the results that you have and try to ascertain whether you have answered your study question to a satisfactory degree. Do you have a story?

A study will always be designed with the aim of answering a scientific question by looking at it from different angles. In the most classic example, an interventional prospective clinical study, the aim of the study would be to learn whether Drug X can cure Disease Y. This is an extremely broad and over-simplified scientific question that would have to be translated into several specific questions. The definition of "curing" the disease will have to be converted into a collection of tangible, measurable outcomes including, for example, results of questionnaires, results of lab tests, imaging procedures, biopsies and other assessments. Each of these is an independent result that sheds light on a certain aspect of the drug's effect on the patient's condition. In addition, in such a study, aspects of drug safety would also be assessed. When reviewing results of such a study, the investigator should ask: How do the results relate to one another? Does one support the other? If results of laboratory tests indicate an improvement, do the responses to the questionnaires indicate improvement in the patient's condition as well? If the results support one another and together point to the same answer, then you are "good to go". If not, you need to assess the degree of discrepancy and try and come up with hypotheses to potentially settle it.

Consider, for another example, a study that is aimed at assessing the effects of certain changes to the parameters of an imaging procedure on its cancer-diagnosis value. It is reasonable that in such a study, you would compare the diagnosis that you achieved with this new imaging technique, to those you got using one or more other diagnostic tools. If the results of the comparisons show that all diagnostic tools provide the same diagnosis, then of course, the results support one another and the paper can be written and published. If, however, the new imaging technique is supported by one diagnostic tool and contradicted by another, then you should carefully consider whether the work is "ripe" enough to be written. Was the study designed and conducted appropriately? What could be a possible explanation for the different results? If you do decide to go ahead and publish at this stage, these points will need to be addressed in the paper.

4.2 How Many Potential Papers Do You Have?

As I mentioned above, the aim of research is answering the scientific question by looking at it from a few different angles. Consider, for an example, a retrospective patient-record study assessing whether non-adherence to the instructions-for-use of a specific medication has any adverse effects on the non-adherent patients. Such a study could ask the following sub-questions:

- What proportion of the patient population falls under the (pre-defined) definition of non-adherence?
- Are there specific characteristics of the non-adherent population (such as demographics)?
- Are there specific medical issues/abnormal laboratory findings/anomalous imaging findings that are statistically correlated to non-adherence?
- Are those findings manifestations of disease exacerbation/relapse?
- Are the findings characteristic of all non-adherent patients, or are they specific to users of a certain brand/dosage form?

These are only a few possible angles from which to analyze this study question and there are many more. However, in this specific set of sub-questions, upon satisfactorily answering questions 1–3, there is enough substance in the study to warrant publication of a paper. The following questions can comprise an independent study that can sustain a separate article.

Certain studies involve the development of a new research method, such as a new questionnaire, a new laboratory assay, a new data-mining technique or others. If the new method is indeed innovative, it is sometimes appropriate to publish it as a separate paper. In some multidisciplinary research teams, the team members that develop the method belong to a non-clinical discipline. If you consider the example of the data-mining technique, the method may be written-up and published in a bioinformatics journal. At the same time, the findings and their clinical implications, may be better suited for a more clinically-oriented journal, and thus can be published separately.

If you have written a thesis, the introduction chapter of your thesis may be adequate as a basis for a review article (see Chapter 5). However, it is a good idea to postpone the writing of this review until all full research articles are well into their submission process. For one thing, it would be very good to be able to cite your own published research articles in such a review, and for another, the review and revision cycles will provide you with a better focus of your entire body of work, making the review article more coherent.

Importantly, consider the aim of the publication. When your immediate goal is to increase the overall number of publications (usually in the earlier stages of your career) on your curriculum vitae (CV), then dividing your work into minimally-publishable-units[1] is warranted and you can target lower-ranking journals for these publications. If, however, you are in a position to aim higher and the ranking of the journal in which you publish is of the utmost importance, it is probably better to try and produce a coherent, rounded work describing the complete study.

4.3 Structure of the Results Section

The Results section of the article should be divided into subsections, preferably, each containing the answer to one of the aforementioned sub-questions. The order of result presentation should be the most logical one. Many times, it is the chronological order in which the study flowed, but this is not always the case. In any study involving a gathering of a sample, be it recruitment of human participants to a prospective clinical study, gathering of medical records for a retrospective study, or

---

[1] https://en.wikipedia.org/wiki/Least_publishable_unit

locating articles for a systemic review, the first sub-section will always describe the actual study sample. In this sub-section, you will note the sample size and its major characteristics. If your actual sample differs markedly from the parameters you have outlined in your Methods section (eligibility criteria, sample size), you should note that in the results, and offer a short explanation.

For example: "*The calculated sample size required for statistical power of XXX, was 10 patients; however, due to extreme weather conditions during the study period that impeded patient arrival at the clinic, we were only able to recruit 5 patients into the study*".

If your study involves different groups (such as treatment and placebo groups, or healthy and diagnosed groups), it is important to point out any major differences between the groups, particularly differences that could potentially have affected the results.

Beyond presentation of the sample, the most important result, which comprises the main answer to the overarching scientific question, should be presented first. If you are reporting results of a study that was conducted based on a study protocol in which the study aims were pre-defined, the first result to be presented is the result of the Primary Endpoint/First Specific Aim. For example, if you conducted a study to evaluate your ability to excise a cancerous mass using a new endoscopic technique, the first presented result would be the percentage of the masses (or their actual size) that was removed with the new technique, as compared to the use of traditional techniques. In another example, in a retrospective study that you conducted to find out whether premature births were correlated to medications taken during pregnancy, the overall number of premature births in your sample would be presented as part of the characteristics of your study population, and the medication found to be associated with premature births would be presented next, as the first and most important result. In the latter example, the following results may be the specific regime/dosage associated, and/or demographic characteristics of the population that experienced this putative adverse effect.

4.4 Visual Aids

Results can be presented in text or with visual aids, including tables, graphs and other types of figures. Some journals provide the option of presenting videos as online-only supplementary materials. Presentation of results in the text should be used only for a very small number of data points or to present qualitative results. Remember that the reading of a scientific manuscript is different than leisure reading and that your readers may skip the text altogether and choose to focus on the visual aids.

4.4.1 *Cross-Referencing*

Do not reiterate the detailed content of your visual aids in the text. The text should be used to provide an overview of the results, point out the most important findings presented in each visual aid and lead the reader through the logical flow of the entire study. It should be used to tie the sub-questions together into a coherent answer to the overarching scientific question of the study. When mentioning a result in the text, always mention the units and include a cross-reference to the relevant visual aid. You can do that at the beginning of a paragraph *"As can be seen in Figure 1..."* or at the end of the paragraph, in parentheses *"(see Table 1 and Figure 3A)"*.

4.4.2 *Visual Aid Structure*

Visual aids should be constructed in a logical manner, usually from left to right and from top to bottom, and you should strive for them to be understandable even by someone who has not read the entire text of the Results section.

Try to focus on presentation of the main results; remember that a very dense figure with a large number of small panels is hard to comprehend and may impede your ability to convey your message. Make sure that any text within a figure is legible even on a printed black-and-white paper version at the actual printed size. While it is true that all materials are available for online reading and the reader can zoom-in, do not count on that. Remember that many times you can provide more details as supplementary materials, and thus not everything has to be presented within the main text body. It has been my experience that figures with up to 6 panels, and tables with up to 6 columns and 12 lines are easy to read and absorb in one take. If you have a very large table with dozens of columns and lines, you can create a smaller table with important findings and present it in the paper, and provide the full table as supplementary material. Do not go to the other extreme, there is no benefit to a table with a single line; this amount of data should be presented as text only. Visual aids or their legends, should always contain clear information about units (see Section 3.2). Make sure to be consistent with units throughout your paper.

4.4.3 *Captions and Legends*

The caption (title) of a visual aid is not its legend. The caption is a concise (no more than one sentence), informative description of the visual aid.

Example: *"Table 1: Demographic and Clinical characteristics of the Study and control groups"*

Example: *"Table 2: Incidence and Odds ratio of developing disease XX in a 10-year follow-up comparing men and women"*

Example: *"Figure 1: mRNA expression of Gene A and Gene B is regulated by Hormone C"*

Example: *"Figure 2: Anti-Cancer Drug XX leads to an increase in overall survival"*

Legends are not usually added to tables. It is sometimes useful to add table footnotes, in which abbreviations and special markings (for example asterisks marking statistically-significant results) are detailed. When relevant, you should mention the statistical test used to obtain a certain result.

The figure legend, in contrast to the figure caption/title, is a more elaborate explanation of the content of the figure. In multi-panel figures, the distinction between panels should appear in the legend. Any use of colors (for example, in double-stained immunohistochemistry images), any markings (such as asterisks, arrows or arrowheads), and any abbreviation in the text within the figure, should be explained in the legend. In figure legends, as in table footnotes, it is advisable to mention the statistical test used to obtain a certain result. It is sometimes appropriate to point out major findings in the legend as well.

Example: *"Figure 1: Experimental setup. Cells or whole tissues were extracted from animals and (A) placed within a liquid suspension, or (B) plated on substrates as a control. The suspension was then incubated in a 25°C humidified chamber for 40 minutes and immersed in complete medium. Cells were either submitted to (C) heat stress or (D) kept as controls. 7 days after plating, cells were analyzed morphometrically for growth. Green arrow points to membrane protrusions. The examples shown are representative of at least 3 experiments. (E) Growth rates by experimental group. *p<0.05 vs. control (Student T test)."*

4.5 Instructions for Authors

Specific instructions for authors (see also Section 2.4) concerning the presentation of results, that you should look for when preparing your manuscript for submission:

- Is there a limit on the overall number of tables and figures?
  This is a major consideration when deciding how many results to present in the current paper.
- What are the allowed dimensions for visual aids?
- What are the technical requirements for images? Make sure you read and understand these requirements. A good resource to help you cope with these requirements is the book *Preparing Scientific Illustrations* (Briscoe, 2013).
- Are tables and/or figure legends included in the overall word count or page count of the manuscript?
- Is there a word count limit on figure legends?
- What is the required format for tables?

- Are literature citations allowed in tables? If so, what is the appropriate format for including a table-citation in the bibliographical list?
- For the submission: should visual aids be included as part of the main document or as separate files? If the former, where within the document should they be inserted (next to the relevant text or at the end under a separate heading)? Where should figure legends be inserted?
- Is there a requirement (or strong suggestion) to upload original data to an online resource?

Beyond the instruction provided to authors by the journal, it is wise to inspect previously-published papers in your target journal that deal with similar subjects. You will get a notion of the conventional way of presenting certain types of results and can adjust your own presentation to match. Presenting data to a reader in a familiar format facilitates understanding.

4.6 Writing Style

The Results section should be written in the past tense and in relatively short sentences. You can choose to use either the active (use the first-person plural) or passive voice, with simple universal terms, avoiding jargon. Abbreviations should be used very sparingly, with the full term spelled out at the first appearance of the abbreviation in the text. It is better to limit yourself to well-known abbreviations and avoid the invention of manuscript- or study-specific abbreviations, no matter how sophisticated it looks to you at first glance. Always remember that the ultimate goal of a scientific paper is to convey the information as clearly as possible, not to dazzle your reader with your writing skills. Inanimate objects (including genes, proteins, tissues and organs) should be referred to in the third person, without any anthropomorphic or possessive terms. Thus, a gene does not "*want to be expressed*" and a protein does not "*attempt to reach the cell membrane*". In another example, instead of writing "*its att site*", write "*the chromosomal att site*". Grammatically, a group of patients is an inanimate object. The group did not "*have a higher blood pressure*" rather "*on average, a higher blood pressure was measured in patients in group A compared to group B"*. Visual aids are also inanimate objects, and thus, while this is a quite acceptable and widely-used sentence structure in scientific publications, my personal preference is to avoid the phrasing: *"Figure 1 shows the results of the first experiment"* or *"The table presents the data"*. I much prefer *"Data is presented in the figure"* and *"Details can be seen in the table"*.

In the Results section, limit yourself to presenting the results of the current study, and do not compare them to previously-published data, not even your own. Do not interpret your results in this section, unless you are writing for a journal in which the sections of Results and Discussion are explicitly allowed (or required) to be combined. It is sometimes acceptable to explain the logic flow between parts of the study, when a result led to the next step of the study.

Example:" Results *of the analysis of the questionnaires administered to children led us to hypothesize that XXXX. To test this hypothesis, we composed the second questionnaire, which we have administered to parents"*.

However, you need to be wary of over-interpreting your results. It is usually preferable to mention any relationship between your findings and others', in the Discussion section (see Chapter 6) and not here. When your study begins with establishing an experimental system through ensuring it conforms to previously-described characteristics, it can be appropriate to say that results were "as expected". For example, in a study looking at the antibody titer in the plasma of patients vaccinated with two different batches of a vaccine, you can say *"As expected, the antibody titer of both groups was markedly increased following the first booster injection; however, the increase was larger among patients vaccinated with batch A compared to Batch B"*. Do not write *"In this experiment, in accordance with the results presented by XX, we saw that..."*. This type of assertion belongs in the Discussion.

Do not offer actual interpretations of your results in the Results section, but do use quantity language to convey your assessment of the magnitude of your results. You can find a wide range of quantity language phrases and terms in the book *Science Research Writing for Non-Native*

Speakers of English (Glasman-Deal, 2009). This should be done cautiously; my personal preference is to always opt for reserved language. Always use language that can realistically be attributed to your actual results. Avoid bombastic adjectives for the description of an effect; very rarely will you see results that merit descriptions such as "a profound effect" or "an extreme difference". It is better to say that the difference was "marked", "appreciable" or "noticeable" because that is a direct reference to the way in which you observe your results.

Example: *"Differences in the mean systolic blood pressure (SBP) between the groups were noticeable as early as 2 weeks after treatment initiation. By Month 2, mean SBP was markedly lower in the treatment group and the difference was maintained throughout the remainder of the study".*

Try to avoid the use of "significant" for anything other than data that has been analyzed statistically and found significant. When reporting clinical results, be sure to use language that conveys whether the results are not merely statistically-significant but whether the magnitude is clinically-meaningful.

4.7 Some Notes on Ethical Result Presentation

The starting point for ethical result presentation is the relevant reporting guideline (see bullet No. 5 under Section 2.4). In addition, you can consider these general ethical principles for result presentation:

1. Whenever relevant, the results of controls should be presented, and in a transparent manner that allows for a real comparison. When presenting laboratory experiments that you have run multiple times, present the results and the controls used during the same run of the experiment and not the best image of a control that you have ever obtained. For example, if you have run a certain Western blot multiple times, your figure should include the experiment and loading control from the same run, on the same day under the same experimental conditions.

   Be extra careful about machine-generated graphs and make sure that the scale used for presenting the controls is the same as the one for the experimental group.

2. Image editing is so easy to do and there are so many possibilities, that it may be hard to know what is an acceptable adjustment to an image for enhancing the visibility of a result, and what may be considered unethical image manipulation. The Rockefeller University Press has established 4 basic guidelines for image manipulation[2] that may help you:

    - *No specific feature* within an image may be enhanced, obscured, moved, removed, or introduced.

    - Adjustments of brightness, contrast, or color balance are acceptable if they are *applied to the whole image* and as long as they do not obscure, eliminate, or misrepresent any information present in the original.

    - The *grouping* of images from different parts of the same gel, or from different gels, fields, or exposures must be made *explicit* by the arrangement of the figure (e.g. dividing lines) and in the text of the figure legend.

    - If the *original data* cannot be produced by an author when asked to provide it, acceptance of the manuscript may be revoked.

3. Transparency is a fundamental principle of ethical writing and it can take many forms. An important aspect of transparency is the ability and willingness to share original source materials. Some examples for source materials are:

    - Original, machine (laboratory equipment/medical device)-generated images

    - Original study protocols

    - Original briefing documents submitted to and letters of approval received from Institutional ethics committees and/or review boards

    - Original, signed informed consent forms

    - Original, machine-generated high-throughput data, including DNA sequencing[3], gene expression, proteome analyses (Perez-Riverol *et al.*, 2015) and others

---

[2] http://www.councilscienceeditors.org/resource-library/editorial-policies/white-paper-on-publication-ethics/3-4-digital-images-and-misconduct/#343ref
[3] See example for DNA sequence submission in https://www.ncbi.nlm.nih.gov/geo/info/

- Original patient files in paper or computerized formats
- Original filled questionnaires
- Original audio- or video recordings of interviews, surgical procedures and others.

You must retain these and other types of source documents in a place that is accessible to you, and file them in a manner that allows easy tracking and identification. A coherent documentation and filing system will allow you to retrieve materials and provide them for review, should the need arise.

5

The Introduction

Chapter 5 in 200 Words for Geniuses

When choosing the literature search engine to use, consider which are available to you, what type of literature you would like to read and cite (articles, books, etc.), and the topic of your study (biomedical, pharmacological, psychological, interdisciplinary). To make best use of it, become acquainted with Pubmed's search features such as the different filters, Related searches and Medical Subject Heading (MeSH).

The logical flow of the Introduction section is from the general to the specific. You start with the general field of research and end with your own study's details. In your Introduction, point out the gaps in current knowledge or the medical unmet need that your research is aimed at filling. Outline your hypothesis, define the specific aims of the study, and explain how they were chosen to meet the need.

When presenting the current status of knowledge, the standard of care/diagnosis, and the unmet need, use the present tense. When describing findings from previous studies, use the past tense. Make sure to present trends and main ideas from previous work. Choose reliable sources of information, preferably primary (original articles) and not secondary sources (review articles, other citing articles).

Make use of citation management software and adhere to the journal's referencing style.

5.1   Search Engines for Biomedical Literature

In Section 1.1, I have provided some tips on how to stay up-to-date with the literature on an ongoing basis. In this way, you will be familiar with the main trends and leading authors of your field of research. Still, after surveying your results and understanding the overarching message that you want to convey in your article, you will need to run a few focused literature searches. There are many scientific journal indexes; they share a lot of characteristics but differ from one another and are each suitable for a different set of uses. A continuously-updated list is available on Wikipedia[1]. There are a few points to consider when deciding which index to use for your literature searches.

5.1.1   *Availability*

First, you need to know which indexes are available to you personally or through your institution's library. Two of the leading search engines that are available for free and are used by researchers in the biomedical sciences are Pubmed[2] and Google Scholar[3]. Other indexing services, such as Scopus[4] and Embase[5], both published by the publishing giant Elsevier are available only with a subscription. PsychInfo[6], published by the American Psychological Association is available through a number of vendors with a subscription and also offers individual paid-use options.

5.1.2   *Types of Literature*

Next, you need to know which types of literature and/or information sources you would like to access.

---

[1] https://en.wikipedia.org/wiki/List_of_academic_databases_and_search_engines

[2] https://www.ncbi.nlm.nih.gov/pubmed

[3] https://scholar.google.com

[4] https://www.elsevier.com/solutions/scopus

[5] https://www.elsevier.com/solutions/embase-biomedical-research

[6] http://www.apa.org/pubs/databases/psycinfo/

PubMed is a service of the U.S. National Library of Medicine; it is the user interface and search engine used to search the Medline database. Pubmed contains 27 million citations, covering all of the Medline database with some additional citations. It is a biomedical and life sciences database that includes only journal articles. Pubmed is part of the Entrez series of databases of (among others) online books (quite limited), genes and proteins. It is very important to understand that Pubmed searches in a human-curated database. Curation is done by literature review committees at the journal level; journals are included in the database based on scholarly criteria. Furthermore, the indexing by human librarians includes tagging the articles for important content information, including whether an article is a review, whether it reports on a clinical trial, whether the study was conducted on humans, which gender and age groups, all of which are extremely useful for focusing your search (see below).

Embase is also focused mainly on the biomedical sciences, but it offers a much more in-depth coverage of drugs and pharmacology and hence is a better resource for studies on topics of pharmaceuticals, including pharmacovigilance and drug development. It currently includes 32 million citations encompassing all of Medline and many additional journals, mainly from Europe. Unlike Pubmed, it provides citations from conference abstracts in addition to journal articles.

Scopus is an interdisciplinary index that covers, in addition to biomedical journal articles, titles from physical sciences, social sciences and humanities. The Scopus index includes over 54 million citations of journal articles, books, book chapters, and conference abstracts covering all of Medline and Embase in addition to other sources. Thus, it may be useful for studies of an interdisciplinary nature, such as health policy or health economics topics.

PsychInfo is a database of publications in behavioral science, social science and mental health. It covers approximately 3.5 million records, including journal articles, book chapters, books, and dissertations. Studies on a wide range of medical topics including psychiatric studies, pediatric development studies and others, may benefit from literature searches on PsychInfo.

All of the above-mentioned resources index only peer-reviewed publications and they each employ their own selection process for quality prior to including a journal in the index. Thus, they are all good resources to assist in weeding-out sub-par publications from your research. In contrast, Google Scholar is not a human-curated database but a search engine of the whole Internet which narrows the list of results based on machine-automated criteria[7]. It provides results from thousands of different websites and there is no selection with respect to the quality of the journal in which the paper was published. Meta data about the articles, including their exact citation and date of publication, are collected from many sources and the same article may appear twice with slightly different meta-data. Google Scholar searches the entire text of the article, whereas Pubmed searches the title, Abstract and tagging information[7]. Google Scholar provides results from conference abstracts, theses or patent applications, all of which are not good sources of information to cite in your own paper. Google Scholar, by its very nature, is interdisciplinary.

5.1.3 *Full Text of Articles*

Most search engines accessed through your institution's computer system will have links to the full-text of articles that your library has paid for, or are provided under an OA model (see Section 2.1.2). When working outside of an organization's system and in need of papers whose full text is available for free, note that Pubmed only retrieves free full text articles that are included in the PMC archive[8], whereas, Google Scholar may provide access to the full text of an article that is posted on other websites, such as the author's personal website or ResearchGate[9].

Both free search engines are constantly evolving and advancing in their capabilities to provide better and more relevant results. Some studies have found that Google Scholar provides more relevant results to clinical searches than Pubmed (Nourbakhsh *et al.*, 2012; Shariff *et al.*, 2013);

---

[7] http://libguides.lib.msu.edu/pubmedvsgooglescholar

[8] https://www.ncbi.nlm.nih.gov/pmc/

[9] https://www.researchgate.net

however, my personal preference still remains Pubmed for subject searches. I use Google Scholar in a limited way, generally to obtain information about specific papers.

5.2 Tips for Effective PubMed Searching

Pubmed is a multi-faceted tool that can be used in many different ways. There are short, user-friendly tutorial videos on the website's home page that you can view to learn how to use it to best suit your needs. Below are some features that I routinely use.

5.2.1 *Filtering Results*

Pubmed offers many filters to narrow down lists of results. My most frequently used filters are:

- Publication type, when I am looking for review articles
- Free full text
- Publication dates; I prefer current literature and so when my initial list includes more than 10,000 entries, I limit my search to the past 10 years.

As a side note, Scopus and Embase offer a variety of filters as well.

5.2.2 *Related Searches*

On the main search result page, you will be offered other search possibilities, that may be relevant to the topics you are working on. I find that this helps me avoid missing papers that do not have my exact terms in their list of keywords, abstract or title.

5.2.3 *Medical Subject Heading (MeSH)*[10]

Because this is a human-curated database, librarians tag the papers in a way that allows grouping of similar medical subjects together, even

---

[10] https://www.ncbi.nlm.nih.gov/mesh/?term=cancer

when they use different terms (for example: cancer, neoplasm, malignancy, tumor) and vice versa, separate papers that use similar terms in reference to different medical subjects (for example: "bypass surgery" for coronary artery occlusion or for bile duct injury). MeSH headings are organized as "trees" with major and minor subject headings. When you run a general search on Pubmed, by default the search spans all MeSH headings; however, when you limit your search to the most relevant MeSH heading or sub-heading, you will greatly increase the relevance of the papers in your list of results.

As a side note, EmBase also offers the option of choosing topic subheadings manually from a list. Scopus, because it searches a few databases simultaneously, only offers natural-language search options with no option for headings.

5.2.4 *Related Articles*

When opening the page for a specific Abstract, you will be offered related papers, ones that possibly report on similar methods, similar medical topics or similar populations. This is yet another very useful tool to avoid missing papers that do not have your exact terms in their list of keywords, abstract or title.

5.2.5 *Cited By*

Another option available on the page of a specific Abstract is a list of papers that cite it. This is very useful in cases where you are looking at older literature and are interested to know how the field of research has evolved in the ensuing years after its publication. The limitation of this tool is that it only presents citations in papers that are included in the PMC archive. In contrast, Google Scholar collects information on papers citing the one you are interested in from a much wider range of sources. You can see how many papers cited your paper of interest, and open a list of all citing papers. Note that this is not a good tool for bibliometric studies. A much more reliable tool is the Web of Science[11] scientific

---

[11] https://www.webofknowledge.com/

citation index, which systematically collects and indexes the citations of papers. However, this is a subscription-based tool and is only available to researchers working within paying institutions.

5.3 The Structure of the Introduction Section

The logical flow of the Introduction section is from the general to the specific. You start with the general field of research and end with your own study's details. In the eBook: English Communication for Scientists ("Unit 2: Writing Scientific Papers"[12] n.d.) the suggested sub-structure for the Introduction section is: Context, Need, Task and Preparation for text. Below is my take on the suggested content of each of these sub-sections.

5.3.1 *Context*

The first sentences of the Introduction should provide the reader with a frame of reference. What is your paper's field of research? In this sub-section, when relevant, you will provide information about epidemiology, status of current knowledge and standard of care.

As with everything else, the journal is a primary determinant of the structure and content of your Introduction section. As I mentioned in Section 2.1, the journal's "aims and scope" tab can provide you with information about its intended audience. This is important, because you should adjust the content of your Introduction to suit this audience. Thus, you do not need to provide a lot of details about the medical condition you are studying to an audience of experts, but you may need to provide more details about its symptomology and epidemiology to a wider audience that has less expertise in the field.

5.3.2 *Need*

In this sub-section, you should point out the gaps in current knowledge or the medical unmet need that your research is aimed at filling. When writing for an audience of experts, in this sub-section you can outline any

---

[12] https://www.nature.com/scitable/ebooks/english-communication-for-scientists-14053993/writing-scientific-papers-14239285

current debates in the field about best practices and for all audiences mention how, in light of the most recent advances in relevant basic and clinical research, there are still topics to be studied.

5.3.3 Task

In this sub-section, you outline your hypothesis, define the specific aims of the study, and explain how they were chosen to meet the need that was mentioned earlier. For instance, in the case of a prospective clinical study, in this sub-section you would provide information about the product you tested and what led you to hypothesize that it would be appropriate for treating the studied indication. This sub-section is probably going to be citation-heavy; you would need to provide the background that formed the basis of the rationale for your study. You should consider the journal's target audience when writing this sub-section. When you write your paper for a methodology-focused journal, you should provide more technical details here than if you submit a paper reporting the same results to a more clinically-focused journal. Another consideration is your results. The provided background information should lay the groundwork for explanation of your results.

5.3.4 Preparation for the Text Body

Here, you should provide a very general and short description of what you did in the study.

Example: "*This was a retrospective study looking for risk factors for coronary artery disease among persons working in construction and undergoing medical check-ups between the years 2000–2010*".

Another example: "*In this study, we treated mice with various dosages of Drug X and assessed them for liver damage by method Y*".

Some authors find it appropriate to include the highlights of their main results in the last paragraph of the Introduction. Personally, I do not like to do that. I think that the Introduction does not need to include any information about the results.

5.4 Style

In the instructions for authors (Section 2.4) you will learn about any word count limit or page limit for the Introduction. In cases where the word count limit is defined for the entire paper, and there is no specific limit on Introduction length, you should consider allocating most of the volume allowance to the Results and Discussion, and keep your Introduction focused and concise. One way to keep your focus is to limit your review of literature to current (past 10–15 years) publications. This can assist you in avoiding lengthy explanations about the evolution of knowledge in the field from its beginning and up to the point of initiation of your own work.

When presenting the current status of knowledge, the standard of care/ diagnosis, and the unmet need, use the present tense. When describing findings from previous studies, use the past tense. Make sure to present trends and main ideas from previous work, and not a list of "A found this and B found that". The exception is a case in which your current work is a direct continuation of previous work. An example could be long-term follow-up of patients who have previously participated in a prospective clinical trial, or in-depth characterization of protein structure and function following a study that identified a new disease-linked mutation. In such cases, you should go into the details of the methodology and results of the previous study.

If you cite work from your own group, clearly say "we have found...", this is not vanity, it is transparency. Stick to clear language, not heavy on jargon. Use short sentences, although avoid stenographical style and make minimal use of abbreviations.

5.5 References

In a scientific journal article, you can cite only data that have been published in recognized sources, such as scientific journals or books. You should try to avoid citing "soft" information sources such as graduate theses that have not been officially published, patent applications or websites that are not systematically archived. Systematic archiving can be assumed, for example, for official websites of governmental entities, or newspapers. Websites that provide medical information for the general public should not be cited; rather, you should search for the source of information, check it, and if verified, cite the original source. Do not take numerical data directly from review articles or other citing articles; check the source to verify the accuracy. You can cite unpublished data, but only very sparingly (better not more than once in your article) and such data can only be used to support a minor point in your work. It cannot form the basis for your entire study rationale. Conference abstracts should not be cited unless they have been published as part of a volume of proceedings. This is because conference booklets are not available to the general public and not indexed in databases and thus, cannot be considered a verifiable source of information.

Be critical of the articles that you cite. Make sure that the journal is scientifically sound. As I mentioned, using Pubmed as your search engine can provide you with a basic level of confidence that the journal has been assessed by professionals and found adequate for inclusion in the database. After spending some time reading the literature, you will become familiar with leading research groups in your field. Try to base your work and rationale on publications by experts. When you spend a lot of time trying to find an article that supports your ideas or approach and finally find one, prior to citing it, ask yourself "if it was not in support of my work, would I consider it a worthy source of information?"

A citation should appear at the end of a paragraph or following a few consecutive sentences that describe findings from a paper, or a trend of findings from a group of previous papers. You do not need to repeat the same citation at the end of each sentence within a paragraph. Make sure you adhere to the journal's citation style. In general, there are two main referencing styles in biomedical journals: in-text citations numbered by their order of appearance in the article, accompanied by a numbered bibliographical list in the same running order; and in-text citations provided with the last name of the first author and the year of publication, accompanied by an alphabetized bibliographical list. However, each journal has its own variation of citation style which will be detailed, including examples, in the instructions for authors. I strongly recommend the use of automated citation-management software such as Endnote[13] (which now offers a limited free, online option[14]), Zotero[15] or Mendeley[16] (see 5b in Section 1.1). These can automatically insert the citations and the bibliographical list according to a certain journal's style. As they retrieve citation information directly from the databases, it is more accurate than manually copied information. The automated management prevents mistakes such as publications that are included in the bibliographical list, but are not actually cited in the text, or vice-versa, cited in the text but missing from the list. In addition, it is very convenient, especially in cases of numbered citations, to have the software automatically and accurately update the order and numbering of the citations and not have to do so manually. Endnote is proprietary and costs money, journal-specific citation styles are constructed by the manufacturer and available for download from the product website. ZOTERO is an open-source freeware; MENDELEY is owned by Elsevier and operates in a "freemium" model, a certain level of use is free and some aspects of service are subscription-based. They use Citation Style Language (CSL) citation styles that are constructed by users and are available for download either from their respective websites, or from the CSL editor website.[17] Some journals offer links for downloading their specific citation style for either Endnote or CSL software users. When you use user-generated CSL styles, be sure to check the examples provided on the CSL editor website, or the formatting of a single reference you insert into a word document, and make sure that the format adheres to the journal's instructions. In my opinion, when you use "official" styles (such as Endnote or journal-provided CSL styles), you do not need to verify them.

---

[13] http://endnote.com/
[14] http://endnote.com/product-details/basic
[15] https://www.zotero.org/
[16] https://www.mendeley.com/
[17] http://editor.citationstyles.org/about/

6

The Discussion

Chapter 6 in 200 Words for Geniuses

The logical flow of the Discussion section is the opposite of that of the Introduction section: from the specific to the general. You start with your own study's details and end with the general field of research. In the first paragraph of the discussion section, you highlight your main results. You can mention numbers, but aim to provide an overview, emphasizing the most important result and do not repeat everything you already wrote in the Results section.

Next, offer an interpretation of the results. You can make a limited amount of speculation, but do not over- extrapolate.

Place your findings in the context of other studies in the field. If your results are in accordance with previous publications, note that, but also point out in what way your results provide new information. If your results contradict what is currently known, assuming that you are confident your work was done properly and results are valid, offer explanations for the discrepancy.

Acknowledge the limitations of the study. Explain what your methodology can provide valid information about, and what it cannot. Discuss how well your participant population represents the population whose unmet need you wanted to fulfill with your study.

Always provide a concrete conclusion, which is the answer to your research question.

Offer future directions for the research, even those that may not be within your ability to perform.

By far, the hardest part of the paper to write is the Discussion. The reason is that it does not have quite the same level of inherent structure, and the range of variety in style and content is very wide. There are a few recommendations that I can make to assist you in writing this section of your paper, but ultimately, it would depend on your specific work, results and style.

6.1 Give an Overview of your Main Results

The logical flow of the Discussion section is the opposite of that of the Introduction section: from the specific to the general. You start with your own study's details and end with the general field of research. In the first paragraph of the Discussion section, you highlight your main results. You can mention numbers, but aim to provide an overview, emphasizing the most important result and do not repeat everything you already wrote in the Results section. Do not cross reference back to the visual aids you used in the results. Never introduce new data in this section that was not already mentioned in the Results section. In some rare cases, it is appropriate to insert a figure into the Discussion section; such a figure may be a schematic or a flow chart that aids in visualizing a principle or a process that can be deduced from your work.

6.2 Interpret your Results

Next, offer an interpretation of the results. You can make a limited amount of speculation, but do not over- extrapolate. An observation that 3 out of 4 mice show a 20% longer survival with treatment compared to control does not mean that the treatment will extend patients' lives and should immediately become part of the standard of care for the disease. It may, however, mean that this observation suggests a potential effect that warrants further investigation. Likewise, if you conduct a retrospective patient-record study assessing the incidence of respiratory complaints and find that it is higher by 35% in your clinic's patients residing in a certain area, you cannot declare the area unfit for human habitation. However, you may suggest in your Discussion a hypothesis about environmental hazards in that area.

Be extra cautious about what you checked and what you did not. In a retrospective analysis of patient compliance with a home-based treatment regimen, the fact that a higher rate of non-compliance was associated with a specific adverse event may suggest that the adverse event caused the non-compliance. However, unless you conducted a survey and asked patients to provide their reasons for non-compliance, your data do not conclusively prove causality.

6.3 Compare your Findings to Those of Others

Place your findings in the context of other studies in the field. If your results are in accordance with previous publications, note that, but also point out in what way your results provide new information. What does your study add?[1] It may be that your population has yet to be studied, your method is novel or that you have applied a known principle to a new field.

If your results contradict what is currently known, assuming that you are confident your work was done properly and the results are valid, offer explanations for the discrepancy. Be respectful, do not imply that others did not carry out their work correctly or report their results faithfully. Try to understand what could constitute a true scientific reason for the divergent findings. What were the differences between the studies? Population? Conditions? Types of analyses? Instruments?

As I mentioned in Chapter 5; in the Introduction, when citing literature, you should generally, write overviews of trends in earlier research. However, in the Discussion, it is many times appropriate to provide details about specific earlier studies and to compare your current work to each of them.

6.4 Limitations

Acknowledge the limitations of the study. You can do that in a standalone paragraph, or as a continuous flow of text of the Discussion. Explain what your methodology can provide valid information about,

---

[1]See Section 8.4: some journals require you to write a paragraph explaining what is already known and what your work adds.

and what it cannot. For example, a retrospective study showing an increase in the rate of patients presenting with a certain complaint may suggest that it is becoming more prevalent, but it may also indicate growing patient awareness due to information availability. Many research tools such as questionnaires, clinical assessment scales as well as medical instruments have well-known and published limitations. Read about them and try to understand how they apply to your study.

Discuss how well your participant population represents the population whose unmet need you wanted to fulfill with your study. Consider the adequacy of your sample size. Do not apologize or completely invalidate your work; be matter-of-fact and explain how, despite its limitations, your work provides new and worthy information.

6.5 The Conclusion

Always provide a concrete conclusion. The conclusion is the answer to your research question, which you have defined from the outset, and refined as you proceeded through your work. You can note reservations in the conclusion paragraph (e.g. *"Our results, provided they are confirmed in a larger sample size, mean that..."*) but do not resort to empty, meaningless phrases like "In conclusion, our study expands the knowledge in the field", "In conclusion, our study sheds some light on..." if you do not support them by a concrete conclusion.

The conclusion paragraph should be short, no more than a few sentences. Do not re-iterate the results again here, and there is generally no need to include numbers in the conclusion. For any paper reporting on clinically-related work, consider whether the you can make some recommendations based on the results and conclusions. Such recommendations may refer to treatment or evaluation of patients.

6.6 Future Directions

Offer future directions for follow-up studies, even if you do not plan on performing them yourself. This does not mean that you should publicize the next specific aim on your funded grant and provide your colleagues and competitors with ideas on how to scoop you. It means that you can either propose a whole new future direction (*"In the future, it may be interesting to see whether this approach is also adequate for the treatment of other auto-immune indications..."*) or a study that addresses the limitations of your own (*"Future studies looking at this phenomenon could potentially use method XXX, which may offer a more detailed view of ..."*).

7

The Abstract and Title

Chapter 7 in 200 Words for Geniuses

The Abstract should be written once the manuscript is finished, or at least when it is in an advanced state to decrease the chances of a discrepancy between the content of the Abstract and the main body of the text.

Adhere closely to the instructions for authors, especially the Abstract structure and word count. A structured Abstract should contain the following parts: Background, Methods, Results, Conclusion. These suggested parts can serve as a template for writing your Abstract even if it is unstructured.

Dedicate most of the Abstract to your results, and include as many numbers as possible.

The Abstract should mention the main methods only, but do not neglect to mention the statistical methods. Questionnaires, disease rating scales and other such research tools should be mentioned by name.

The Background sub-section of your Abstract should be very short, only 1 or 2 sentences, approximately 10% of the Abstract.

Unlike the main text body, the Abstract does not contain a Discussion section. Write a concise, one-sentence conclusion which corresponds to the conclusion at the end of the Discussion section, only shorter.

Make sure your Abstract contains your key words. Do not include references in your Abstract and try to minimize abbreviations.

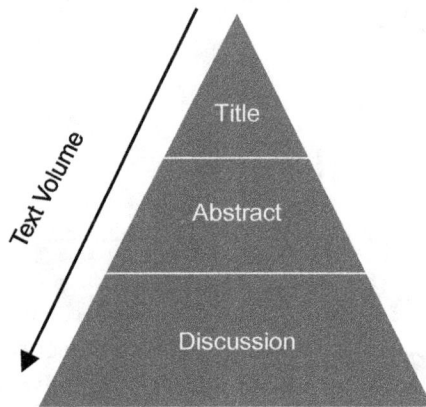

The most important points of the work should appear (preferably in the same order, displaying the same logic), in the Title, Abstract, and Discussion sections of the paper, with an increasing volume of text.

7.1 Writing Your Abstract

The Abstract should be written once the manuscript is finished, or at least when it is in an advanced state. At this stage in the process, you know exactly what your main message is, and the chances of a discrepancy between the content of the Abstract and the main body of the text are much smaller (see also Chapter 8).

Author guidelines include instructions on the size and format of the Abstract. Pay special attention to the allowed number of words for the Abstract. If you do not see a clear word count limit for the Abstract, keep searching throughout the instructions for authors and, where relevant, the online submission web page. Shortening an Abstract is not merely a technical process and converting a 300-word Abstract into a 200-word one, requires thought, may require debate among co-authors and can be time consuming. It is very rare to have an unlimited space for the Abstract, and there is no flexibility, the online submission system will not allow you to insert an Abstract that exceeds the word count limit. Be sure you know the requirements and abide by them, so you do not get stuck in the submission process.

Some papers require a structured Abstract, whereas others require a single paragraph that is not structured. In the absence of other instructions[1], a structured Abstract should contain the following parts: Background, Methods, Results, Conclusion. These suggested sub-headings can serve as a template for writing your Abstract even if it is unstructured. In such cases, the template helps you avoid omitting important information and you can adjust the wording later, to provide the text with a better flow.

7.2 The Content of the Abstract

7.2.1 *The Results Sub-Section*

The vast majority of your readers will only read the Abstract, so it should convey the most important points, your results. The importance and centrality of the results should be translated into the proportion of volume they take up in the text of the Abstract. My suggestion is to use 50% of the allowed number of words in the Abstract for the results. Use numerical results and as much actual data as possible in the Abstract; this widens the exposure of your findings and may increase the likelihood of your paper being cited. Of the entire set of your study results, present the most important one (the one that is the answer to your research question) first. Survey your results and choose which are meaningful enough to be presented in the Abstract. It is okay to leave some less-important results for presentation only in the main text body, but be transparent. Do not present only the "good" results (those that support your hypothesis) in the Abstract. Be extra careful not to present any result in the Abstract that is not included in the main text body.

Example I: *"Of the 100 enrolled participants, 59 (25 women and 34 men) comprised the safety analysis set. Mean (SD) exposure to study drug was 28.3 (11.8) days; cumulative exposure duration was 12 days or longer in*

---

[1]One example of an elaborate and strict Abstract structure is the one required by the *British Medical Journal* (*BMJ*): Objective, Design, Setting, Participants, (Interventions), Main outcome measures, Results, Conclusions. See: http://www.bmj.com/about-bmj/resources-authors/article-types/research/editors-checklists

57.4% of participants. A total of 50 participants (84.7%) reported treatment-emergent adverse events (TEAEs) (TEAEs leading to treatment discontinuation, 15 [25%]; severe TEAEs, 4 [6.7%]; serious TEAEs, 1 [1.7%]). TEAEs reported in greater than or equal to 10% of participants were headache (13.2%) and upper respiratory tract infection (11.4%). Elevations in systolic blood pressure for longer than 5 days were observed in 5 subjects (8.5%), and elevations in liver function tests were noted for 3 subjects (5.08%)."

Example II: "*Patients reported a considerably higher HrQoL than their caregivers on the QoL, EQ-5D, and EQ VAS (p < 0.001). Higher disease severity groups showed significantly worse results in HrQoL. The mean self-reported QoL decreased from 30.2 ± 4.6 in the group with the lowest severity scores to 20.1 ± 6.5 in patients with the highest severity scores (p < 0.001). A considerably lower HrQoL was shown for hospitalized patients compared to outpatient settings (proxy-rated QoL 17.6 ± 4.4 versus 27.0 ± 8.1, p < 0.001). Depressive symptoms, and reduced functional capacity were evaluated for their impact on patients' HrQoL. Multivariate models explained between 12% and 24% of the variance in patients' HrQoL.*"

7.2.2   *The Methods Sub-Section*

For research papers that are not focused on methods, the Abstract should mention the main methods only. You should avoid minute methodical details in the Abstract, but do not neglect to mention the statistical methods you used. The Methods sub-section should be approximately 25% of the allowed number of words in the Abstract. For the very least, it should be clear (where applicable) which species were studied, whether the study was clinical or basic, prospective or retrospective. Well-known methods can be mentioned by name only. Questionnaires, disease rating scales and other such research tools should be mentioned by name; however, even in the Abstract, this may not always be sufficient. You may need to provide a very short explanation about what type of information you collected with each research tool you used.

Example I: "*Health-related data on 2000 adolescents (11–19 years-old) examined in the hospital between January 1st, 2010 and December 31, 2012 were analyzed to derive non-Hodgkin's Lymphoma (NHL) incidence up to December 31, 2012. Cox proportional hazards modeling was used to estimate the hazard ratio for NHL associated with demographic and medical history parameters.*"

Example II: "*Cultured rat cells were treated with culture medium (control group), Substance AA at 100 µM (Substance AA group), Substance XX at 10 µM (Substance XX group), and Substance AA plus Substance XX (Substance AA + Substance XX group), respectively. The oxidative stress, mitochondrial membrane potential (ΔΨm) and apoptosis of the cells were evaluated by a series of assays, including ELISA, flow cytometry, immunofluorescence microscopy and Western blotting*".

7.2.3 *The Background Sub-Section*

The Background sub-section of your Abstract should be very short, only 1 or 2 sentences, approximately 10% of the allowed number of words in the Abstract. In it, just provide the reader with the most immediate context for you study. The background sub-section of the Abstract is usually not the place to go into debates in the field, unless your current study was aimed specifically at resolving such a debate. Do not refer to previous work in the field unless the current work is a direct follow-up (or rebuttal) of that work; just provide a frame of reference for your project in broad terms.

Example I: "*The purpose of this study was to find groups at a higher risk for suffering from cerebrovascular accidents among residents of assisted living facilities in Arizona*".

Example II: "*Scaffolds may have enhancing effects on cellular growth in engineered tissue models*".

Example III: "*There is an unmet need for an easy and cheap measurement of the effects of braces on the alignment of the spine in patients suffering from scoliosis*".

7.2.4 *The Conclusion*

Unlike the main text body, the Abstract does not contain a Discussion section. In the Abstract, you do not compare your results with those of other groups (again, unless this was the stated purpose of the study) and, it is generally not expected of you to elaborate on the limits and caveats of your findings in the Abstract.

Write a concise, one-sentence conclusion to your Abstract. It should correspond to the conclusion at the end of the Discussion section, only shorter. The two locations of the conclusion in the paper cannot be different and definitely cannot contradict each another.

As I mentioned in Section 6.5, avoid empty phrases such as: "*Conclusion: This study provides insights into the regulation of Hormone BB homeostasis at the transcriptional level and provides a better understanding of the potential impacts of Substance XX on the thyroid endocrine system of vertebrates*". Instead, write a definitive (even if qualified) conclusion and stand firmly behind your results: "*These results suggest that Substance XX promotes the secretion of Hormone BB through effects on the WWW Transcription factor and can form the basis for future studies of this potential endocrine disruptor*".

While not always applicable, my personal preference is to mention any potential applications for implementation of the study results. For example, consider an Abstract of a paper describing the validation of a new assessment method, that found that the method is reliable and results reproducible over a wide-range of different parameters. My suggestion for the conclusion of this Abstract is "*These results prove that our method is very reliable and can potentially be adopted as part of routine clinical evaluations of patients with the diagnosis of YY*".

7.3 Writing Style for the Abstract

Make sure your Abstract contains your key words; this will cause it to appear higher on the list of search results in Pubmed and other search engines.

Do not include references in your Abstract and try to minimize abbreviations. The Abstract should be widely understood outside of your field; try to avoid the use of jargon. Write clear, concise sentences and convey as much of the most important points while abiding by the word count limits set by the journal.

7.4 The Title of the Article

Ideally, the title should be written when the article is completely ready for submission. Obviously, this could not be the case, as the title is chosen right at the beginning of the writing process. However, when the writing process is done, it is important to re-visit the title and make sure that it is still adequate. Many things can change over the process of working on a paper (see Chapter 8). Sometimes the focus of the paper changes, because you decided to divide the work into two papers and the result you referred to in your original title is no longer a part of the current manuscript version you are submitting. Sometimes during the work on a paper, your research has advanced and a newer and stronger result should take the spotlight.

Remember that the title of your paper is the one thing sure to be read by anyone whose search results include your article. Reading your title is the first interaction with your work and thus the title should convey the most important point, in a clear manner. The title of a scientific article is not like the title of a newspaper article; it should not be phrased in an intriguing manner for the purpose of coaxing people to read it. The main finding should be clearly stated right at the top of the paper.

Your audience is wide, and may vary in their proficiency in English. To ensure clarity, use plain English and provide as much information as is possible within the title wordcount limits. Do not use puns or word-play, don't try to be "cute". I also recommend against phrasing an article title in the form of a question.

Example: Instead of writing: "*Does hunger promote secretion of acid in the stomach?*", use: "*Hunger may promote the secretion of acid in the stomach*".

Many research fields have typical styles and structures for article titles. Having chosen your target journal, read through some of its issues' tables of contents and try to adapt your title to match the style of previously-published papers in the journal.

8

When You Have a Full Draft

Chapter 8 in 200 Words for Geniuses

Have your work scientifically-reviewed on an ongoing basis and editorially reviewed at advanced writing stages.

Establish the order of the authors prior to initiating the writing. Define a document "owner" (usually the first or last author) who will be responsible for coordinating the writing and review through to publication.

Use American English or UK English consistently as per the journal's instructions. Check that abbreviations are used consistently and are spelled-out in full at first mention. Make sure that the bibliographic list is consistent with your in-text citations, and all are adherent to the journal's citation style.

The Title Page should contain: Article Title; Author names, highest academic degrees and affiliations; Corresponding author contact details; Wordcount, table and figure counts; Key words; Running title; Statement of conflict of interest.

The letter to the editor is the place for you to explain the importance and merits of your study, and why it may be of interest to the journal readership. Do not copy large sections of your Abstract into the letter.

When asked to recommend potential reviewers for your paper, recommend researchers from the same field, from your own or another country.

Use the same order and spelling of your names across all your publications. An ORCID is recommended.

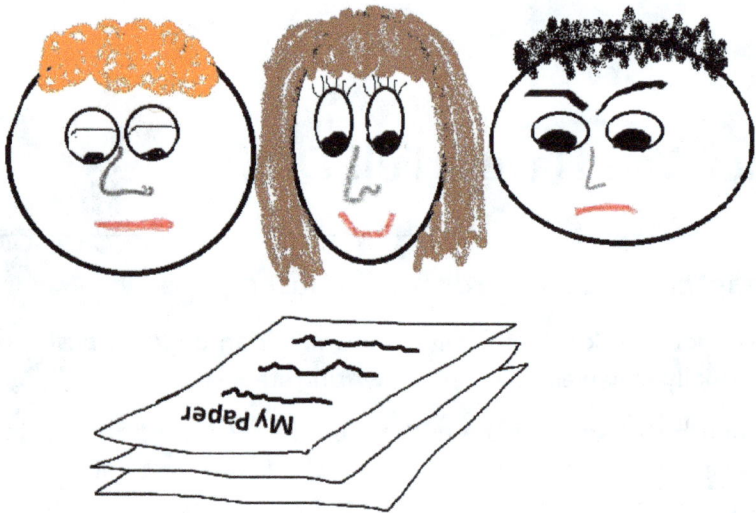

A scientific paper goes under several rounds of review and revision before it reaches its final, published form. Prior to submission, it will be reviewed by your colleagues and supervisor, as well as paid editors and proofreaders (if available). After submission, it will be reviewed by the editor and peer-reviewers. Finally, after acceptance, it will be reviewed by production professionals.

8.1　The Two Types of Pre-submission Review: Scientific Review and Editorial Review

When you have written a full draft, or a substantial part of it, it is time to have it reviewed. There are always several layers of review that each document should undergo. If you are lucky enough to be working with a mentor, he/she should be your first reviewer and should be involved with the writing work from an early stage. In the absence of such a function in your professional life, seek input from senior colleagues, preferably people who have already published scientific papers. The types of input you should seek can be grouped into two main categories: the Scientific and the Editorial, each encompassing several general types of questions.

- **Scientific Review**

  Does the reviewer agree with the way you conceptualized your research question?

Does the reviewer agree with the way you designed your research and the methodologies you chose in order to answer the research question?

How does the reviewer evaluate the way you carried out your research? What is the assessment of the execution of experiments and other types of research procedures?

What is the reviewer's assessment of the actual study sample (be they clinical study participants, animals used in experiments, articles used in a meta-analysis, etc.), is it robust in terms of size, adherence to study eligibility criteria, representation of the general population, etc.?

- **Editorial Review**

In the reviewer's opinion, is your writing easily understood?

Do your major points come across clearly?

How does the reviewer assess the level of your English writing? Are there many spelling and grammar mistakes?

Is your use of abbreviations correct and consistent?

Are your cross-references to visual aids correct?

Are the captions and legends of your visual aids clear?

Do your sections "work together"? Is there a description of the method for each result described?

The Scientific review is an ongoing process. You should continuously seek this type of input and advice, in the early stages from your mentor and close senior colleagues, and at later stages, from co-authors and collaborators (see Chapter 8.2). The Editorial review can wait till the later stages, when the manuscript is in an advanced state. This type of input should be sought from people who are more proficient in English than you, have more experience in writing and publishing scientific papers, but not necessarily as well-versed in your scientific topic. These could be colleagues at your own scientific/academic level who are not involved in your research, or professional, paid editors and proof-readers.

8.2 Notes on Writing a Scientific Paper With Multiple Co-authors[1]

Current research is very rarely done by a single investigator and thus a scientific paper almost always has multiple authors. Writing an article with multiple collaborators can be chaotic and time consuming. However, if you adopt a few of the principles that underlie document writing operating procedures used by pharmaceutical companies, the process can become much simpler as well as faster.

The below-described processes can help greatly if adopted by all writers. However, even if some or all of these principles are adopted only by the sub-group of authors that are most involved in the project, the writing process can be easier.

8.2.1 *The Owner of the Article*

The order of the paper's authors and any special circumstances such as "co-first" authorship, should be discussed and agreed upon prior to initiating the writing.

As the reader of this book, you are most likely either the first author of the paper, or the last author, meaning you are the mentor or group supervisor for the project. If you are either of these, then you are most likely the article's "owner" (see below). You should strive to hold some type of process-initiation meeting (in person, by telephone or online) during which several decisions can be made:

- First, if this has not yet been decided, the article's "owner" must be determined. This author can be, but does not have to be, the first author. The meaning of article ownership is that the author is responsible for coordinating the writing and review activities of the various

---

[1] Adapted from my blog post: https://www.sciencewriteright.com/single-post/2016/06/14/Managing-the-writing-of-a-multiauthor-paper

authors within the group as well as for external activities such as taking care of professional editing and proof reading, professional statistics services, submission to the journal and communication with the editorial office until the article's publication. For this reason, this author should be the corresponding author.

- The group needs to decide how independent the article owner can be, and to what extent other co-authors wish to be involved in making strategic decisions for this publication. For example — in case of a rejection from the first submission target journal, is there a need for a joint discussion in order to decide on the next submission destination, or can the article owner submit sequentially to as many target journals as may be necessary to get the article published? Can the owner independently decide on further analyses at the request of reviewers?

8.2.2 *Areas of Responsibility*

After the article owner has been chosen, areas of responsibility need to be defined. Who should be responsible for writing each section? Sometimes, these will be obvious, such as in a project that is a collaboration between a clinician, a statistician and the head of a genetic research laboratory. Here, it is clear who writes each part of the Methods and Results sections. In most cases, the article's owner or the first author (if they are not the same person) will be responsible for the survey of literature and writing the Introduction. However, interpretation of the results and deciding on the structure and content of the Discussion may not be as obviously assigned.

8.2.3 *Work Process Including Timelines*

Finally, the hardest part is making the decisions pertaining to the work process. As I mentioned above, each group member should indicate how involved in the writing process they want to be. Some will want to write specific sections and some would prefer just to review and offer comments.

If you are writing with a group that is not located in the same geographic region and does not communicate outside the context of co-authoring the paper, if possible, it is advisable to schedule a series of joint meetings to discuss the article in advance.

It is important to know what the preferred mode of communication is for the group and for each collaborator, and what is the best way to communicate with them in order to receive rapid responses. A convenient solution worth considering, is storage of data (including drafts of the article) in an online repository accessible by everyone in the group[2].

It is very important to try to get the co-authors (or at least some of them) to commit to timelines of reading and reviewing of drafts. You can inquire of any prolonged absences of the co-authors. In terms of the process, it is very useful to hold rounds of review and revision sequentially, so that each contributor is able to see the input provided by the people who have done the reviewes earlier and you would not have to consolidate the comments of various reviewers from several separate drafts. For the sake of this process, it is best when notes are provided in "Track changes" mode, with the reviewer's identity and time of review.

As the article owner, you should keep track of drafts, when and to whom they were sent and who returned comments. When you have established a long co-writing collaboration with a group, it may be appropriate to institute delivery of reminders to those late in providing input and group updates about the status of each article until its final publication.

8.3 Finalizing your Paper and Preparing it for Submission

8.3.1 *Proofreading*

After you have the final draft of the paper and the content has been reviewed with both types of review mentioned above, you (or a paid

---

[2] For example https://www.box.com/home or https://www.google.com/drive/

professional editor/proofreader) should run a technical proofreading round on your paper.

- **Spelling and Grammar**

  The abilities of word-processor spelling and grammar checks keep evolving and improving; make smart and informed use of them. Teach the machine your field's vocabulary, but make sure you are teaching it correctly — confirm the correct spelling of professional words as they appear in scientific articles in your field.

  You can also use dedicated proofreading software, such as Grammarly[3] or Ginger[4] or others, that can help you identify grammar and spelling mistakes. Some of those offer add-ons to your word processing software and can run the proofreading on your document without the need to copy all of your text into their websites. However, you need to be cautious with implementing their suggested revisions, as such programs are not primarily designed to meet the needs of scientific writers.

  The spelling should be consistent. Check the requirements of your target journal with respect to the type of English for your manuscript. Some journals, based on their official location will define whether you should write in American English (mostly, American journals) or UK English (some European journals); however, for most journals the requirement is only to maintain consistency throughout the manuscript. For a large part of the text, choosing the correct spell checker from your word-processing software, would be enough to identify mistakes. But, you need to manually check scientific terms that are not included in your spell-checker's dictionary, and make sure that they are spelled correctly (with respect to the type of English) and consistently throughout your document; including tables, figures and figure legends.

  Do not alter the wording of the references in your bibliographical list, as these are a part of the cited article's digital identity and

---

[3] https://www.grammarly.com
[4] http://www.gingersoftware.com/

should remain as provided to your citation management software by the article indexing service (see Section 5.1).

- **Abbreviations**

As I mentioned before, abbreviations should be used very sparingly, with the full term spelled out at the first appearance of the abbreviation in the text. After the first mention, you should only use the abbreviated form, apart from section and sub-section headings. So, when proof-reading your final draft, make sure that abbreviated terms are spelled-out in full only upon their first mention in the main body of the text.

There is a professional proofreading tool called PerfectIT[5]. It offers a host of proofreading functions, most of which are more useful for people who proof read professionally and are less relevant to a person proofreading just their own work. However, the tool has a very reliable abbreviation-analysis function that may prove useful, especially if you are writing a big, text-heavy manuscript such as a review article.

Note that the Abstract is a stand-alone mini document and thus, an abbreviation needs to be spelled out separately upon first mention in the Abstract and then again upon first mention in the main text. Make sure that the use of abbreviations is consistent and that different terms that have the same abbreviation are not both abbreviated the same way in the document (e.g. BM for bone-marrow and for body-mass in the same manuscript), because this may be confusing to the reader.

- **Cross-references**

Check to make sure that all references from within the text to visual aids are correct and do not need to be updated. If the instructions for authors allow submission of visual aids within the same file/document, then this can easily be ensured through the use of the cross-reference function of your word processing software, which is updated automatically[6]. If you are submitting the visual aids as separate files,

---

[5] http://www.intelligentediting.com/
[6] As an example, instructions on creating an automatically-updated cross-reference in MSWord software https://support.office.com/en-us/article/Create-a-cross-reference-

you should manually check each cross-reference for accuracy. In addition, when you cite a number from a visual aid in your text, make sure that it is consistent with the number that appears in the visual aid.

- **References**

  You need to make sure that the bibliographic list is consistent with your in-text citations; do all of the references you cite in your text appear in your list and nothing else? In addition, ensure that your style of referencing adheres to the journal's instructions. As I mentioned in Section 5.5, the best way to avoid mistakes in referencing, is to use citation-management software.

8.3.2 *Ensuring Adherence to Instructions for Authors*

Throughout this book (most detailed in Sections 2.4 and 4.5) I have repeatedly emphasized the importance of adhering to the journal's instructions for authors. When you are getting ready to submit, it is important to check one last time that your manuscript is in complete compliance. While I am sure you paid attention to requirements and made an effort to write the paper accordingly throughout your work process with respect to content, now is the time to deal with formatting issues.

A few formatting points to check for compliance, and my suggestions for the default choice in case you checked and did not find specific journal instructions:

- **Line Spacing**

  By default, use double-line spacing.

- **Numbered Lines**

  By default, do not number your lines.

- **Document Headers and Footers**

  By default, do not include headers and footers in your submitted documents, because during the step of the submission process in which your document will be rendered to PDF, the system will create its own headers.

  The exception to this is page numbers. By default, number your pages at the bottom of each page.

- **Section and Sub-section Headings**

  By default, do not number headings, and use 13/14 points bold face black fonts for section headings and 12 points bold face black fonts for sub-section headings.

- **Images**

  By default, do not paste images into your word-processing document; submit them as separate image files, named by their manuscript designation (for example: "XXX *et al.*, Figure 1").

  Make sure you understand and adhere to technical requirements such as file formats and image resolutions (see Section 4.5).

- **Tables — Location and Format**

  By default, paste tables into your word-processing document and do not submit them as separate files.

  Insert tables at the end of the document, following your reference list, especially if they require a landscape page layout.

  By default, do not use vertical lines in your tables and do not shade any cells. Use bold face font for the column headers, and align the text to the center of each column.

  Do not use paragraph breaks in tables, only manual line breaks.

- **Word and Other Item Counts**

  Make sure you adhere to word count limits, and verify whether there are separate limits for specific sections (especially the Abstract; see

Section 7.3). Be sure not to exceed the allowed number of visual aids or references.

- **Anonymity**

  By default, include author names below the title in the document that contains the Abstract and main text body.

  Some journals require that you anonymize your manuscript completely (see Section 9.2); in such a case you should save the Title Page and main text as two files, remove any author-identifying information from the document containing the main text, and include it only on your standalone Title Page (see Section 8.4).

8.4 The Title Page

These days, the submission of every scientific journal article is accompanied by a separate Title Page. This is a technical document that is checked by staffers at the editorial office, that are not professionals in the journal's scientific topic area, and are not editors, members of the editorial board of the journal or peer-reviewers.

Each journal's instructions will include a section on what should be presented on the Title Page. Below is a list of components that are generally requested.

- **Title (See Section 7.4)**
- Author names

  Make sure *you can justify* the authorship of each person included in the list of authors (see Section 1.5) and that the order of authors has been agreed-upon (see Section 8.2).

- Author highest academic degree
- Author affiliation

  Be sure to verify each co-author's most up-to-date affiliation with him/her, including institution, department and address.

- Author contact details

  Make sure you have current contact information for each co-author, as you may be required to provide it, even if not within the Title Page itself. Editorial offices many times send out messages to all co-authors requesting confirmation that the author is aware of the submission and had approved it. Make sure that all your co-authors are aware that you have submitted to a certain journal and do not object (see also Section 8.2).

  As mentioned before, the document owner should be the Corresponding Author. The full name, highest academic degree, mailing address, e-mail address, and telephone and fax numbers of the document owner should be provided in a separate small paragraph under the heading Corresponding Author.

- Word/character count, table and figure counts

  Make sure you count the words on the very final draft, the version that you submit.

- Key words

  Always use the entire allowance for key words. With the exception of Google Scholar (see Section 5.1) that searches the entire available text of an article, search engines use the Title, Abstract and list of key words in their searches. The richer your list of key words, the more likely your article is to be included in the list of results for a given search. Include the main terms from your article and, if more words are allowed, add terms from the wider field of your research. Note that hyphenated terms (for example "blood-sugar") are usually counted as a single term, whereas individual words are counted separately.

- Running/Short title

  From your full title, remove redundant words so that you adhere to the character-count limit set by the journal, but be sure that the resulting title is still meaningful and clear.

- Disclosure statement of conflict of interest for each author and research funding sources.

  Understand and adhere to the format requirements for the disclosure (see Section 1.4).

State any funding that supported the study, including scholarship grants to students whose work is being presented. Provide grant numbers when available.

8.5 The Letter to the Editor

The letter to the editor is many times perceived as a marginal thing that gets written at the end of the process, with minimal exertion. This approach is adequate when the paper has very clear advantages and qualities that make it perfectly suitable for publication in the target journal. However, if the paper is not quite what the journal normally publishes, or when the paper is not reporting on very high-impact work, such as reports of negative results or reports on studies conducted on very small sample sizes, then the letter becomes more important and you need to dedicate more time and effort to it.

The editor reads the letter alongside the Abstract and so there is no logic in copying large sections from the Abstract to "fill" the letter. The letter is the place for you to explain the importance and merits of your study, and most importantly, why it may be of interest to the journal readership. Recall the parameters that led you to choose this journal as a submission target (see Chapter 2) and what in the journal's "aims and scope" made you think it would be a good fit for your paper. Use this logic as the basis for the text of your letter.

The letter may also be the place to communicate some things about the paper or the study that are not mentioned in the paper itself. Such, for instance, you may note in the letter a name of a prospective reviewer that you request not to review your paper, for reasons of potential conflicts, etc. In another example, if the data had been presented in a conference or in a paper in a non-biomedical journal, then you should mention that in the letter as well.

8.6 Suggesting Potential Reviewers

Some journals invite authors to recommend prospective reviewers for their manuscripts (see Section 9.2). In such cases, you may be tempted to recommend your best friend as a reviewer. Of course, this is unethical (unless he/she just happens to be a renowned expert in your field), and in any case, there are rules to these recommendations. Usually, the number of reviewers you will be invited to suggest is 3. Some journals specify a limit on how many of them may be from your institution, and some journals also limit the number of recommended reviewers from the authors' own country. This type of policy follows recent scandals, in which people recommended their friends and even themselves as reviewers[7].

So, who should you recommend? Use the maximal number of allowed reviewers from your institution. For the external ones, your best choice is a researcher from the same field, preferably from another country, with whom you (or your boss/mentor/senior colleague) have had previous collaborations but is not involved in the current work. If there is no one like that, survey your article's bibliographical list. From the papers that are directly related to your study's topic, use the newest papers, those whose authors are most likely to still be working in the field. Of those, you can recommend either the first or last authors as potential reviewers for your work.

Do not copy the contact information from the cited paper and forward to your target journal without checking. Look the person up, make sure they are still affiliated with a reputable academic institution, and try to provide the most accurate and up-to-date contact information. Contacting such a person and requesting their permission to recommend them as reviewers may seem like the courteous thing to do, but it may also be perceived by the reviewer and/or the journal as an attempt to break the masking of the review process and a breach of ethical conduct, so I recommend against it.

8.7 The Online-submission Process

Nowadays, submission of scientific articles to journals is done through specialized online submission systems such as those based on the

---

[7]https://www.nature.com/news/publishing-the-peer-review-scam-1.16400

ScholarOne Manuscripts[8] or Editorial Manager®[9] platforms or those of Elsevier-published journals that are based on the EVISE®[10] platform. You, as the author, upload your manuscript and provide its meta-data to the editorial office in a pre-constructed format that helps all stake holders: the authors, the editorial office and the reviewers, to track the process from initial submission to final decision and/or publication (see Chapter 9).

As I mentioned in Section 8.2, the owner of the paper is responsible for submitting the paper and thus should preferably be the corresponding author. Before you start your submission process, you need to make sure that you have the manuscript in final format, all accompanying documents including the letter to the editor, any stand-alone files of images or tables, the Title Page (if it is separate), declarations of conflicts of interest (if they are separate from the Title Page) and current contact information and affiliations of all co-authors. For this latter topic, an Open Researcher and Contributor ID (ORCID; see Section 8.7.1) number is very useful. Other types of information that you want to have prior to initiating the submission process is a list of names and contact information of people you would like to propose to the editor as potential reviewers for your paper (see Section 8.6), a clinicaltrials.gov (or equivalent) number, if applicable, and sometimes, when the journal is the official publication of a professional association of which you are a member, it may be good to have the membership number (member ID) accessible.

The user-interface of these systems takes the shape of a series of online forms with fields you fill with text based on the provided instructions. Usually, the first thing you would be requested to do is create a user name and password for yourself; these credentials can either be journal-specific or, in the case of EVISE, applicable to all Elsevier-published journals. In either case, the same credentials can be used to log in as an author or as a reviewer.

---

[8] http://scholarone.com/products/manuscript/
[9] http://www.ariessys.com/software/editorial-manager/
[10] https://www.elsevier.com/editors/evise

Once you have logged in, you will start the submission process by providing author and co-author information. I find this stage to be a bit frustrating, especially when co-authors are already registered users in the systems, as people tend to define their affiliations differently between their own different publications and mostly differently than the way their colleagues, who have submitted their information to the same system in the past, have done. For example, a doctor may define himself as affiliated with the "*So-and-So institution for the study of childhood cancer, department of pediatrics, Royal hospital of country XXX*" and a colleague, working in the exact same place would define the affiliation as "*Royal XXX hospital, department of pediatric oncology*". The system, not being a human, will log those as two different institutions and this may be confusing and may impact the presentation of affiliations on the paper and the Title Page.

In my experience, most other parts of the submission user interface on all platforms are quite self-explanatory and user-friendly. If you encounter a field that you are not sure how to fill and would like to consult with your colleagues, for example, on the most appropriate topic and sub-topic designation for your paper, you can always save your work and return to it when you have all the necessary information.

Certain systems for certain journals are more flexible, collect some meta-data and then allow the upload of user-generated documents for the rest. Others are stricter, and require the pasting of a lot of information, including the letter to the editor and the Abstract into the form fields, allowing the system to stop the process if the text exceeds the allowed number of words or deviates from the instructions in another machine-detectable way. At any rate, provided you are equipped with all the necessary submission materials and necessary information, the process should take no more than an hour or two.

8.7.1 *An Important Note on Author Identification*

You always want to get credit for all the articles that you have published. But, listing them on your CV is not enough. You want to make sure that when others search databases, they get the complete list of your publications. For this reason, you must write your name in exactly the same way on every submitted manuscript. This means, that you cannot change the spelling of your name in English from one manuscript to the next, you have to make sure that the order of your names (first, middle, last/family) is uniform across submissions to different journals and the use of any initials should remain the same across all publications. However, during a long (and hopefully, fruitful) career, your name may change. For example, I published my first paper a few months before my marriage, and had to do so under my maiden name. Nowadays, if anyone were to search for my name on Pubmed, they would not find this first publication. Another problem is that names are not unique. ORCID[11] is a potential solution to all of these problems with author IDs. It is a code comprising 16 letters and numbers, which is unique to you. You can easily and quickly get one on their website. During the online submission process of your paper, the system will provide you with the option of linking your publication to your ORCID, and if you choose to do so, you will be re-directed to a website for authentication (Haak *et al.*, 2016). While the integration with Pubmed is still in its infancy, it is rapidly growing. As of mid-2017, close to 200,000 publications on Pubmed included authors' ORCIDs, and that number has grown from only about 20,000 in 2015. In January 2016, some publishers and scientific societies have declared that they will start requiring the use of an ORCID[12]. ORCID numbers are not-proprietary, unlike commercial IDs such as the SCOPUS ID (which is now integrated with ORCID). They are also universal, and thus are not as limited in usefulness as specific institutional or national IDs. The vision is that in the future, each author will have their own unique ID so that all, and only their own publications will be linked. Ultimately, readers will be able to search by ORCID and find only the relevant results.

---

[11] https://orcid.org/

[12] http://www.sciencemag.org/news/2016/01/journals-solve-john-smith-common-name-problem-requiring-author-ids

9

Following Submission

Chapter 9 in 200 Words for Geniuses

The journal's decision-making process comprises a technical assessment of the submission, and a content evaluation by the editor and peer reviewers. The final decision is made by the editor.

Peer review, which is either open (all parties are named), single-masked (authors are known to reviewers, reviewers are anonymous) or double masked (all parties are anonymous), yields one of the following answers: "accept as submitted", "minor corrections needed", "major corrections needed" or "reject".

When revising a paper, prepare a Response Document, in which you will address each point in the reviewers' comments, each with the exact location of the change within the manuscript. Try to identify points raised by more than one critic. Those notes will probably need to be addressed even if the article will eventually be submitted to another journal. Try to implement as many suggestions as possible and explain respectfully the ones that you cannot or choose not to implement. For the latter, provide a scientific reasoning, preferably backed by literature.

Make sure you understand the publishing agreement prior to signing it, and specifically your rights.

Review proofs meticulously but limit your changes to those allowed at the proofing stage. Take actions to enhance your paper's visibility online, but verify your sharing rights before distributing the full-text.

9.1 The Decision-Making Process in a Scientific Journal[1]

The process of decision making in various journals is not uniform and is very much dependent on the size of the editorial staff. However, the most important thing to understand is that in every journal, the editor decides whether to publish or reject an article and not the peer-reviewers.

The process can generally be divided into the following steps:

The first step in the process is technical. A staff member, usually not a scientific/medical professional, reviews the submission and makes sure that it meets all of the journal's technical requirements. Currently, electronic submission systems (see Section 8.7) allow staff to discover errors very quickly. Too many words in the article or Abstract, too many tables or images, lack of contact details of the co-authors, incorrect format of citations or bibliography, can all be identified quickly with a superficial review of the submission and the article can be returned to the author for corrections. The staff member must also make sure that the article meets the most basic ethical requirements such as information on the informed consent procedure, approval by institutional review board, and declaration of any of the authors' conflicts of interests. When relevant, they can check that you have provided sufficient details concerning recommended reviewers. Sending the article back to the author at this point is not considered a rejection, and the author can easily correct any such technical errors and resubmit. Nevertheless, this is an unwanted delay in the time until publication and you should strive to avoid it by following the journals instructions for authors (see Sections 2.4, 4.5 and 8.3.2) meticulously.

At the second stage, the article is reviewed by an associate editor, a junior editor (in large journals), or the senior editor (smaller journals). At this stage, the editor checks the article, decides whether it falls within

---

[1]This chapter has been adapted from a post on my blog https://www.sciencewriteright. com/single-post/2016/1/26/The-DecisionMaking-Process-in-a-Scientific-Journal

the journal's scope (see Section 2.1), and critically assesses the content. Following this round, the editor can reject the article or send it out for peer review (see Section 9.2). Rejection at this stage is often a final rejection. If you get a note from the editor saying that your paper does not match the journal's aims and scope or that the editor did not find your paper to contribute sufficiently new scientific information, it means that you are not invited to correct and resubmit. In such a case, you should choose another target journal (see Section 2.3).

The third stage is peer review in which reviewers can recommend either "accept as submitted", " minor corrections needed", "major corrections needed" or "reject" (see Section 9.3).

The last step — reviewer recommendations are sent to the editor and the editor or editorial board makes the final decision whether to accept the article (with or without a requirement for changes) or reject it.

In most cases, when you log into the online submission system (see Section 8.7), you can see the up-to-date status of your paper. There will be an indication on your author page as to whether the editor has the paper, whether it has been sent for peer-review, and whether review has been completed. If there is no such indication, or if the process seems to not be advancing at a reasonable pace (for instance, if the paper is under review for a few months), you can try and contact the staff at the editorial office, or the publisher's customer service to try and find out what is going on.

9.2 Peer Review[2]

I hope you agree with me that someone should check an article before it is published in a scientific journal. If so, who? The journal editor is one person, with a limited capacity and defined areas of expertise. Thus, peer review meets the need for a group of people who have a large

---

[2] This section has been adapted from a post on my blog https://www.sciencewriteright. com/single-post/2015/02/26/Peer-review-like-democracy-is-perhaps-the-worst-method-except-for-all-the-others

enough capacity and wide enough range of expertise to assist the journal in making decisions about manuscripts.

In its ideal form, peer review should be a system in which a group of scientists, with a high level of knowledge relevant to the research in question, read the article carefully, attempt to verify some of the results and exercise impartial discretion in deciding to publish only the most-worthy articles.

The reality is far more complex. The editor sends the article for review by people with expertise in the subject of the article or in related fields. The choice of reviewers can be based on the editor's acquaintance; however, journals have difficulties maintaining relationships with many experts in a large variety of fields, so many times they have to rely on the recommendation of the authors (see Section 8.6). Articles are usually sent to two or three reviewers that may have only remotely related expertise. When reviewers disagree, the article is usually sent to another reviewer in hope that their recommendation will facilitate a decision.

The peer review system suffers from a lot of shortcomings. There are reviewers who agree to review, but then delegate the task to a subordinate with very rudimentary relevant knowledge. Like you, reviewers are very busy and critically-appraising other people's work is almost always assigned a low priority. Reviewers spend a short, condensed time reviewing or worse, read articles sporadically, a minute here and a minute there, and in the mishmash of distractions purport to formulate balanced and thorough opinions.

No one really expects a reviewer to try and repeat experiments. No one has the extra time or resources for that and this type of work could never be funded. So, a reviewer should rely on their experience and prior knowledge to assess your study results and decide whether they seem plausible to them and whether your results, as presented together, make sense. This can partially account for cases of publishing fake results, as sometimes appear in science news.

Although all of us engage in science due to some level of idealism, what level of saint would you have to be to approve the publication of an article by a colleague that you do not like? How about a competitor who you would allow to scoop you by your mere approval? The issue of impartiality is addressed, to some extent, through the practice of double-blind or double-masked review.

Reviews can take one of three forms with respect to transparency:

- Open review: All parties are named. The authors submit the manuscript under their full names with their affiliations, and reviewers sign their reviews. Some of these reviews are even published alongside the criticized articles. A 2-year experiment conducted by a few journals published by Elsevier seems to indicate that open review offers benefits to both authors and reviewers. It compels reviewers to take extra care with their written reviews, to strive for clarity in their comments and to strike an encouraging and constructive tone in their criticisms. It seems to also promote further discussion on the papers[3].
- Single blind/single-masked review: The authors' identities are known to the reviewers; however, the reviewers remain anonymous. This is the most prevalent paradigm for peer-review of biomedical-sciences articles. Under this traditional structure, reviewers can freely express their opinions, without worrying about ramifications from the authors. This is especially important when working in small scientific fields, in which you are likely to know your reviewer. By remaining anonymous, the reviewer can be sure that you will not reject one of his papers in the future, impede his ability to get funded or reject his candidacy for a position, as revenge for harsh criticisms of your work.
- Double-blind/double masked review: The identities of both parties are known only to the editor. In addition to the protections provided to the reviewers, this paradigm is hypothesized to protect authors from bias. It should prevent reviewers from formulating an opinion about the work based on the authors' names and affiliations.

When authors are not named, reviewers would presumably not be affected by preconceptions about the quality of research performed in certain geographic areas or academic institutions, or by certain

---

[3] https://www.elsevier.com/reviewers-update/story/innovation-in-publishing/is-open-peer-review-the-way-forward

demographic groups. While double-masked review is a solid idea, it is limited by its practicalities. To participate in such a review process, authors should purge all identifying information from their paper. This does not only mean submitting a version of the manuscript without the line of author names and affiliations, authors should scrub the manuscript of any hint of their identity. This includes any reference to the institution in which the study was conducted (e.g. *"the study was approved by the IRB of St. Christopher's Hospital"*) as well as any reference to the authors' previous work (e.g. *"we have previously reported similar findings in a different group of patients (Roberts et al., 2010)"*). This is hard to do, requires reviewers to work on a version that would later change so that the identifying text can be re-introduced, and impractical, as, inevitably, especially in small research fields, reviewers are able to guess who the authors are (i.e. which research group) or at least create a narrow list of candidates.

9.3 The Different Types of Reviewer Responses

Answers received from scientific journals can be divided into four main categories: "accept as submitted", "minor corrections needed", "major corrections needed" or "reject".

9.3.1 *Accept as Submitted*

The first, "instant acceptance" is rarely encountered. Each professional in the fields of science and medicine has a unique set of emphases and sensitivities. The chances that a group of three reviewers absolutely agree with the authors on both the scientific substance and the presentation form, are very low. Hence the need to form a ranked list of submission targets and not have just one (see Section 2.3).

9.3.2 *Reject*

There are two main situations in which a journal will reject an article without allowing the authors to correct and resubmit: first — the editor or the reviewers think that the article does not fall within the scope of the journal, and the second — critics think that the level of work is inadequate for the journal. When the reason for the rejection is a mismatch between the subject matter and the scope of the journal, there is probably not much point in arguing, and it is better to invest the time and effort in submitting to another journal, without changing the article significantly. In such cases, the editorial staff may offer an alternative journal within the catalogue of the same publisher (see Section 2.3.3).

If the reason is dissatisfaction with the level of work, it is very important to go through the reviewer comments in detail and understand what they did not like. It is important to use their comments to improve the article before submitting it to another journal, even if, the latter is ranked lower (see Section 9.5).

9.3.3 *Minor or Major Corrections Needed*

Editors interviewed in the British *Guardian*[4] encouraged authors who receive revise-and-resubmit decisions from journals to not be discouraged, to improve their paper and resubmit. In my experience, the scope of requested changes should be a significant factor in the decision whether to implement them. When the reviewers suggest improvements in the writing style, presentation of results, discussion points, etc., it is relatively easy to correct and resubmit. In such situations, it is sometimes possible to seek assistance from a more senior colleague or a professional who had previously published on similar scientific topics to broaden the range of background reading or deepen the discussion.

When reviewers ask for more results, you should check how easy it is to acquire them and evaluate how much time and resources you will need in order to meet the recommendations of the reviewers. Are reviewers asking for a new analysis of data that you already have? Do you need to get new data? Do you or your co-authors have access to the necessary information? For example, when the article describes a clinical trial, do you have access to the medical records of the participants? Is it possible to ask participants to come for another study visit in order to obtain

---

[4] http://www.theguardian.com/education/2015/jan/03/how-to-get-published-in-an-academic-journal-top-tips-from-editors

additional data? Could there be any ethical issues with the actions required to acquire the additional data?

9.4 Revising Your Paper

A scientific journal decision letter usually consists of two main parts:

- The editor's notes with the current decision, and;
- Comments of the peer-reviewers.

It is hard to calmly address criticisms leveled against an article into which you have poured your blood, sweat and tears, but this is the only way to get through the difficult process of publication. In an instructive lecture given by Dr. Jaap van Harten[5], a senior publisher at Elsevier, he gave excellent advice to listeners: set the response letter aside and read it a few days later, (presumably) after the waves of outrage have subsided.

My suggestion is to deal with reviewer comments one step at a time:

First, copy all the text received from the reviewers into a clean document, to be used as a Response Document, and divide it into separate bullet points. Following each point, leave room for your responses.

All revision work should first be done on this separate document, and then implemented into the article text. Try to identify points raised by more than one critic. Those notes will probably need to be addressed even if the article will eventually be submitted to another journal (see Section 9.5).

Below you can find tips for responding to common types of reviewer comments.

9.4.1 *Comment: Missing Information in the Article*

If the information is indeed missing, add it (assuming that the information is available to you) even if when you wrote your paper, you considered this information to be unnecessary for the readers. In the Response

---

[5] https://www.linkedin.com/in/jaap-van-harten-9846b98b/?ppe=1

Document, note that the requested information was added and direct the reviewer to its location in the article (by section and line number. For example: "*The average age of patients in group B was 34± 2 years. This information has been added to the manuscript in the Results section, Line number 4*"). You should not argue and declare that the information is unnecessary, or that it may be confusing. However, if you are unable to obtain the requested information, you can explain in a respectful way, with quotes from literature, why the work supports the conclusion even in the absence of the requested information.

If the information is already in the article, examine the way the information is presented to make sure it is clear, and try to find places in the article in which you can add references to this information. In the Response Document, note that the information exists within the article and direct the reviewer to its location. In addition, you should mention that the presentation of the requested information has been clarified and references added. You should not leave the subject unaddressed and only refer to the location within the article. Try to refrain from responding: "*The information is already in the article, see the Methods section, line 63*". It is certainly a very bad idea to write "*Had the reviewer read the article more carefully, he/she would have noticed...*"

9.4.2 *Comment: The Sample Size is Too Small*

You probably already thought long and hard about your sample size, and a reviewer comment is not the first time you encounter the notion that your sample size is inadequate. However, if you are not in a position to increase the sample size and feel that it is justified, the explanation for sample size selection in the Methods section should be expanded, including quotes from the literature. In the Response Document, you should go into even greater detail to discuss and justify your sample size. You should mention that the explanation in the article body was expanded and provide the location to the reviewer. You should avoid answers such as: "*recruitment for this type of trial is very difficult*" or "*this type of experiment is very expensive.*" A potentially better alternative to the former, is a paragraph on the prevalence of the studied indication, showing that there are not enough available potential study subjects.

The justification must be as scientific as possible. Of course, you should not write "*had the reviewer any experience in this type of research, he/she would know that...*"

If the sample size is indeed too small, you can add text to the article and Response Document which positions the research as "a pilot study" or "a proof-of-concept study" and qualify the conclusions with the need to show similar results in a larger sample.

9.4.3 *Comments: Missing Important References, Stylistic or Grammatical Errors in the Article, Graphs / Images are not Clear*

You should try to fix each point separately as the reviewer requested, and perform a global process of editing and proofreading of the text. There is no need to specify each language and style revision in the Response Document, and therefore, you do not need to implement every single change of this type suggested by the reviewer. You should state in a general way that the article has been revised according to the reviewer's guidance. It is not advisable to argue about stylistic points and raise linguistic or other justifications that your style is correct and the reviewer is wrong. If a reviewer requests that you cite a particular article, you should do so, and indicate that it was done in the Response Document. When the request includes changes to graphs/figures, you should not adamantly defend your design. If there is someone who does not understand what you mean, it might actually be necessary to revise the figure for the purpose of improving clarity. In cases where figures were revised, include the revised version within the Response Document.

9.4.4 *Comment: Results are not In-line with the Reviewer's Own Knowledge and Background Information*

If it is possible to check the reviewer's comments against the literature, do so, and address the articles cited by the reviewer (and other relevant ones) in the Discussion section of your article and within the Response

Document. You should attempt to offer possible ways for resolving the apparent contradictions. You should not underestimate the importance of the works cited by the reviewer or raise suspicions about their findings. Address the comments in a practical and sensible manner.

9.4.5 *Comment: There are Flaws in the Design or Performance of the Study*

In the Response Document, and perhaps within the Methods and Discussion sections of the paper, you should justify the choice of the methodology as an appropriate means for studying the research question (including literature citations). If possible, add information that could better reflect the study conduct, in a manner that addresses the reviewer's concerns. It is helpful to acquire the assistance of a professional (e.g. a statistician) to address such comments.

Even if the reviewer's comments indicate a lack of knowledge or understanding, you should not respond aggressively. You should provide the necessary background information for understanding the method and its specific use in your study. If different reviewers give contradictory recommendations, you can (respectfully) use the arguments of one reviewer to respond to requests made by the other reviewer.

Despite all the advice to keep calm and to the point, sometimes reviewers can go too far, sometimes you can identify that a reviewer is a professional rival or competitor of one of the authors or that a reviewer is operating under irrelevant considerations. In such situations, before deciding to submit to another journal, you can try to contact the editor directly, explain the problem and ask for a round of review with another team of reviewers.

9.5 Revising Your Paper in Case of Submission to an Alternative Target Journal

If you decide to submit to another journal, it is still very important to go through all the reviewer comments, understand them, and see how you can improve the article in order to increase the chances that it is accepted in your next target journal. Sometimes, it is possible to implement only some of the reviewer comments before submitting to another journal. This is especially true if there is a large difference in IF between the first and second targets (see Section 2.3). Keep in mind that there are only a few leading researchers in a specific scientific field, and there is a chance that the editor of your next target journal, will send your article again to the same reviewer. In such a situation, the submission of the article without any substantial change may provoke the reviewer to reject it.

As in the initial submission, read the instructions for authors thoroughly and understand exactly how your paper needs to be adapted to the requirements of your new target journal. If your new target journal happens to be published by the same publisher, it may deviate only slightly from the first in its stylistic requirements. But, if it has a lower IF, this may be due to a smaller, more niche readership (see Section 2.1.1), and this may require adjustments to the Introduction (see Section 5.3) and Discussion (see Chapter 6) of your paper.

9.6 After Acceptance

Congratulations! Your paper has been accepted for publication!

In some academic settings, an official letter of acceptance is enough for you to list the paper on your CV as "accepted for publication in Journal XXX", even if a digital object identifier (DOI) has not yet been assigned.

9.6.1 *Fees*

Following official acceptance, if your paper is to be published in an OA journal and you have not qualified for a waiver (see Section 2.1.2), you will be requested to pay the publication fee. If your paper is to be published in a subscription-based publication, there may still be fees, such as color-page fees, which you will be required to pay.

9.6.2 *Publishing Agreement*

Publishing agreements and copyright are a vast and complicated issue, way beyond the scope of this book. Having said that, I still strongly advise you to understand the agreement prior to signing it, and if you cannot understand it by yourself, enlist the assistance of an experienced colleague or better yet, a legal professional from your academic or clinical institution. Moreover, some publishing houses provide you with several options from which it is your job to choose, making it much more important to understand the differences, and how they affect you with your set of unique circumstances.

General information on this topic is provided by a few of the big publishing houses, Elsevier[6], Springer[7], Wiley[8] and Taylor and Francis[9].

There are a few main points that you need to be clear about, which will affect how your article is handled in the future.

First, you need to understand who owns the copyright to the paper. Under some types of agreements, you retain the copyright, and with others, the copyright is transferred to the publisher or to the academic society that owns the journal.

Second, you need to understand what type of uses of the material will be allowed in the future, and by whom (including yourself). This includes a whole range of uses from reading the full text, to using text and/or visual aids in future publications. The latter can be academic publications such as review articles or books but they can also be commercial materials such as white papers or even advertisements. The use can be commercial or non-commercial.

9.6.3 *Approving Proofs*

After your paper has been accepted for publication, production process will commence. Proofs will be sent to you for your approval, usually accompanied by a list of queries. The format of the proofs can be a PDF

---

[6] https://www.publishingcampus.elsevier.com/websites/elsevier_publishingcampus/files/Guides/U_Pub_Process_brochure_web_042115.pdf

[7] https://www.springer.com/gp/authors-editors/journal-author/journal-author-helpdesk/open-access-/1298#c1272

[8] https://authorservices.wiley.com/asset/photos/licensing-and-open-access-photos/How_to_sign_an_article_license_Author_Services_Feb_2017.pdf

[9] http://authorservices.taylorandfrancis.com/publishing-agreements-your-options/

file that you can add comments to, or a link to an online-proofing system, in which the queries are embedded within the text, and you can add your answers into a hyper-linked list of queries. The latter has the advantage that it will automatically prevent you from finalizing the proofing process if you missed a query and have not answered all of them.

When you read through the proof, do not confine yourself to the list of queries. Go over the entire document in detail and make sure that every word is written correctly, and every number is exactly as you provided it in your submitted version. Pay close attention to cross-references, make sure that the text refers the reader to the correct visual aid for the paragraph or to the correct bibliographical citation. Go over every item in your bibliographical list and check it for accuracy (make sure no errors such as the wrong article by the correct author were introduced during production). If the journal provides links to Pubmed in the bibliographical list, check each and every one of them to make sure they work and are correct. If, during this process, you discover an error that was originally made by you on your submitted version and has not been caught by yourself or the reviewers, you need to notify the editorial office and/or the production team; however, you may not be able to do so directly within the proofing platform.

Very limited changes are allowed at the proofing stage. Those are only technical changes, such as typo corrections, cross-reference errors and similar. You are not allowed to make substantial changes such as re-writing whole sections, adding new/improved results to existing tables or changing the list of authors. If you wish to make this type of change, you need to contact the editor and discuss it with him/her.

9.6.4 *Online Publication and Increasing Your Paper's Visibility*

Usually, once you have approved the proofs, your paper will be published online and assigned a DOI. If you have published in a Medline-indexed journal, the paper will be listed on Pubmed as "Epub Ahead of

Print". At this point, you can claim your paper as published and list it on your CV.

As I have mentioned in Section 2.1, your target journal's IF gives you a very general notion about the level of exposure you can expect for your article. Other pieces of information may also be important, such as the journal's connections to the general media and other publicity efforts they make.

There are some actions that you can personally take in order to achieve better visibility for your paper. This includes posting a link to it on social media and reporting about it to organizations you are affiliated with, that publish newsletters, such as your alumni association. Some papers may justify the involvement of your institution's public relations office, if there is one. Also consider whether the paper may be of interest to any patient advocacy organization.

Making people aware that you have published is always recommended. Providing the full text of your article, however, is a different matter. Most journals provide a few complimentary printed copies to the authors, but in the current era, online availability is much more important.

Prior to posting your full article onto your research group's website or to social media, check your publication agreement. The International Association of Scientific, Technical, and Medical Publishers (STM), has published a consultation for Voluntary principles for article sharing on scholarly collaboration networks ("Voluntary Principles for Article Sharing on Scholarly Collaboration Networks" 2015). The latter does not refer to social media geared specifically toward scientists such as ResearchGate.[10] Rather, it refers to large, sometimes international groups that are involved in an active research collaboration. These groups can include, among others, academics, commercial entities and general public representatives. Those are very loose general principles that mainly state the commitment of publishers to facilitate such sharing without impeding their own rights. A few publishers have policies for what they term "responsible sharing", that explain in general terms what is allowed under specific types of agreements. Elsevier's policy can

---

[10] https://www.researchgate.net

be found online in a few places[11], Wiley's policy is explained here[12] and Springer-nature provides information about their policies here[13].

There is also an online search engine that allows you to find information about sharing possibilities for a publication, based on its DOI[14]. If you are not sure, contact the editorial office and ask them specifically about your paper and what your rights are.

---

[11] https://www.elsevier.com/authors/journal-authors/submit-your-paper/sharing-and-promoting-your-article
[12] http://olabout.wiley.com/WileyCDA/Section/id-826716.html
[13] https://www.springer.com/gp/open-access/authors-rights/self-archiving-policy/2124
[14] http://www.howcanishareit.com/

10

Abbreviations and Terms

10.1 Glossary of Abbreviations

APC	Article Processing Fees
BMI	Body Mass Index
BMJ	British Medical Journal
CONSORT	Consolidated Standards of Reporting Trials
CSL	Citation Style Language
CV	Curriculum Vitae
DOI	Digital Object Identifier
ICMJE	International Committee of Medical Journal Editors
ILAR	Institute for Laboratory Animal Research
IRB	Institutional Review Board
MeSH	Medical Subject Heading
NCBI	National Center for Biotechnology Information
NHL	Non-Hodgkin's Lymphoma
OA	Open-access
ORCID	Open Researcher and Contributor ID
PDF	Portable Document Format
PMC	Pubmed Central
RCT	Randomized Controlled Trials
SBP	Systolic Blood Pressure
SI	from French: *Système international d'unités*
STM	Scientific, Technical, and Medical
TOC	Tables of Contents
UPDRS	Unified Parkinson's Disease Rating Scale
VAS	Visual Analog Scale

10.2 Index of Terms

References

Aggarwal, Rakesh, Nithya Gogtay, Rajeev Kumar, and Peush Sahni. 2016. "The Revised Guidelines of the Medical Council of India for Academic Promotions: Need for a Rethink." *Indian Journal of Urology : IJU : Journal of the Urological Society of India* **32** (1): 1–4. doi:10.4103/0970-1591.173117.

"AMWA–EMWA–ISMPP Joint Position Statement on the Role of Professional Medical Writers." 2017. *AMWA Journal* **32** (N1). AMWA.org.

Briscoe, Mary H. 2013. *Preparing Scientific Illustrations: A Guide to Better Posters, Presentations, and Publications.* 2nd edition. Philadelphia, PA: Springer.

Conners, C. K. 1997. "Technical Manual for the Conners' Rating Scales-Revised." *North Tonawanda (New York): Multi-Health Systems.*

Dunn, W. 1999. "The Sensory Profile Manual." *San Antonio, TX: Psychological Corporation.*

Frank, Martin. 2013. "Open but Not Free--Publishing in the 21st Century." *The New England Journal of Medicine* **368** (9): 787–789. doi:10.1056/NEJM p1211259.

Glasman-Deal, Hilary. 2009. *Science Research Writing for Non-Native Speakers of English.* 1st edition. London ; Hackensack, NJ: Imperial College Press.

Goetz, Christopher G., Stanley Fahn, Pablo Martinez-Martin, Werner Poewe, Cristina Sampaio, Glenn T. Stebbins, Matthew B. Stern, et al. 2007. "Movement Disorder Society-Sponsored Revision of the Unified Parkinson's Disease Rating Scale (MDS-UPDRS): Process, Format, and Clinimetric Testing Plan." *Movement Disorders* **22** (1): 41–47. doi:10.1002/mds.21198.

Haak, Laurel, Paul Donohoe, Véronique Kiermer, Helen Atkins, John Lees-Miller, and Craig Raybould. 2016. *ORCID iD Throughput in Publishing Workflows.* National Center for Biotechnology Information (US). https://www.ncbi.nlm.nih.gov/books/NBK350150/.

Hessmann, Philipp, Greta Seeberg, Jens Peter Reese, Judith Dams, Erika Baum, Matthias J. Muller, Richard Dodel, and Monika Balzer-Geldsetzer. 2016. "Health-Related Quality of Life in Patients with Alzheimer's Disease in

Different German Health Care Settings." *Journal of Alzheimer's Disease : JAD* **51** (2): 545–561. doi:10.3233/JAD-150835.

National Research Council (US) Institute for Laboratory Animal Research. 2011. *Guidance for the Description of Animal Research in Scientific Publications.* The National Academies Collection: Reports Funded by National Institutes of Health. Washington (DC): National Academies Press (US). http://www.ncbi.nlm.nih.gov/books/NBK84205/.

Nourbakhsh, Eva, Rebecca Nugent, Helen Wang, Cihan Cevik, and Kenneth Nugent. 2012. "Medical Literature Searches: A Comparison of PubMed and Google Scholar." *Health Information & Libraries Journal* **29** (3): 214–222. doi:10.1111/j.1471-1842.2012.00992.x.

Perez-Riverol, Yasset, Emanuele Alpi, Rui Wang, Henning Hermjakob, and Juan Antonio Vizcaíno. 2015. "Making Proteomics Data Accessible and Reusable: Current State of Proteomics Databases and Repositories." *Proteomics* **15** (5–6): 930–50. doi:10.1002/pmic.201400302.

Ray, Sumantra, Sue Fitzpatrick, Rajna Golubic, Susan Fisher, and Sarah Gibbings, eds. 2016. *Oxford Handbook of Clinical and Healthcare Research.* Oxford Medical Handbooks. Oxford, New York: Oxford University Press.

Shariff, Salimah Z., Shayna Ad Bejaimal, Jessica M. Sontrop, Arthur V. Iansavichus, R. Brian Haynes, Matthew A. Weir, and Amit X. Garg. 2013. "Retrieving Clinical Evidence: A Comparison of PubMed and Google Scholar for Quick Clinical Searches." *Journal of Medical Internet Research* **15** (8): e164. doi:10.2196/jmir.2624.

"Unit 2: Writing Scientific Papers." n.d. In *English Communication for Scientists.* Nature publishing group. http://www.nature.com/scitable/ebooks/english-communication-for-scientists-14053993/118519636.

"Voluntary Principles for Article Sharing on Scholarly Collaboration Networks." 2015. International Association of Scientific, Technical, and Medical Publishers (STM). http://www.stm-assoc.org/2015_06_08_Voluntary_principles_for_article_sharing_on_scholarly_collaboration_networks.pdf.

www.ingramcontent.com/pod-product-compliance
Lightning Source LLC
Chambersburg PA
CBHW050631190326
41458CB00008B/2226